Praise for *The PlantPlus Diet Solution*

"Eat these words! Dr. Borysenko's personalized PlantPlus approach is a major step forward in cutting through dietary confusion, increasing nutritional literacy, and enjoying true food and good cooking. Joan gets us back on track in a way that's fun, economical, and easy to stick with for the long run."

— **Andrew Weil, M.D.**, *New York Times* best-selling author of *Healthy Aging* and co-author of *True Food*

*"**The PlantPlus Diet Solution: Personalized Nutrition for Life** is the best book in years on nourishing not just your body but your mind and spirit as well. This is a superb example of the integration of cutting-edge science, psychology, and common sense. If the endless stream of diet books makes you want to run in the other direction, **The PlantPlus Diet Solution** is for you. I never thought I'd see a book on nutrition that is fun to read, but here it is. Bravo, Dr. Borysenko, for reminding us that the kitchen can be a sacred site."*

— **Larry Dossey, M.D.**, author of *One Mind: How Our Individual Mind Is Part of a Greater Consciousness and Why It Matters*

"Practical wisdom, crystal-clear science, and step-by-step guidance in using food as medicine from one of the great pioneers of mind-body medicine. This is a terrific book, one to read and savor."

— **James S. Gordon, M.D.**, author of *Unstuck: Your Guide to the Seven-Stage Journey Out of Depression* and founder and director of The Center for Mind-Body Medicine

*"Blending mind and science, Dr. Joan Borysenko establishes the brain-green connection as she creates a New Nutritional Normal in **The PlantPlus Diet Solution.** Her recipe for success combines a simple, flexible, and tasty cuisine, as well as a host of mental tools to stay on track with healthy eating and self-care. She should know, as she lives her message!"*

— **Pam Peeke, M.D., M.P.H., F.A.C.P.,** *New York Times* best-selling author of *The Hunger Fix, Body for Life for Women,* and *Fight Fat After Forty*

THE
PLANT PLUS
DIET
SOLUTION

ALSO BY JOAN BORYSENKO, Ph.D.

Books

Minding the Body, Mending the Mind

Guilt Is the Teacher, Love Is the Lesson

On Wings of Light (with Joan Drescher)

Fire in the Soul

Pocketful of Miracles

The Power of the Mind to Heal
(with Miroslav Borysenko, Ph.D.)*

A Woman's Book of Life

*7 Paths to God**

A Woman's Journey to God

*Inner Peace for Busy People**

*Inner Peace for Busy Women**

Saying Yes to Change (with Gordon Dveirin, Ed.D.)*

Your Soul's Compass (with Gordon Dveirin, Ed.D.)*

*It's Not the End of the World**

*Fried: Why You Burn Out and How to Revive**

Audio Programs

*Reflections on a Woman's Book of Life**

A Woman's Spiritual Retreat

Menopause: Initiation into Power

*Minding the Body, Mending the Mind**

*The Beginner's Guide to Meditation**

It's Not the End of the World (five-part seminar)*

Video Programs

*Inner Peace for Busy People**
*The Power of the Mind to Heal**

Guided-Meditation CDs

*Invocation of the Angels**
*Meditations for Relaxation and Stress Reduction**
*Meditations for Self-Healing and Inner Power**
*Meditations for Courage and Compassion**

*Available from Hay House

Please visit:

Hay House USA: www.hayhouse.com®
Hay House Australia: www.hayhouse.com.au
Hay House UK: www.hayhouse.co.uk
Hay House South Africa: www.hayhouse.co.za
Hay House India: www.hayhouse.co.in

🍃 🍃 🍃

THE PLANT PLUS DIET SOLUTION

Personalized Nutrition for Life

JOAN BORYSENKO, Ph.D.

HAY HOUSE, INC.

Carlsbad, California • New York City
London • Sydney • Johannesburg
Vancouver • Hong Kong • New Delhi

Copyright © 2014 by Joan Borysenko

Published and distributed in the United States by: Hay House, Inc.: www
.hayhouse.com® • *Published and distributed in Australia by:* Hay House Australia Pty. Ltd.: www.hayhouse.com.au • *Published and distributed in the United
Kingdom by:* Hay House UK, Ltd.: www.hayhouse.co.uk • *Published and distributed in the Republic of South Africa by:* Hay House SA (Pty), Ltd.: www.hayhouse
.co.za • *Distributed in Canada by:* Raincoast Books: www.raincoast.com • *Published in India by:* Hay House Publishers India: www.hayhouse.co.in

Cover design: Steve Williams • *Interior design:* Riann Bender

Library of Congress Cataloging-in-Publication Data

Borysenko, Joan.
 The plantplus diet solution : personalized nutrition for life / Joan Borysenko,
Ph.D.
  pages cm
  ISBN 978-1-4019-4148-2 (hardback)
1. Nutrition--Popular works. 2. Diet therapy--Popular works. 3. Self-care,
Health--Popular works. I. Title.
 RA784.B6387 2014
 613.2--dc23
                          2014011697

Hardcover ISBN: 978-1-4019-4148-2

10 9 8 7 6 5 4 3 2 1
1st edition, September 2014

Printed in the United States of America

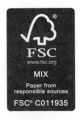
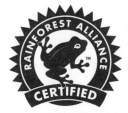

To Gordon Dveirin,
husband, partner, friend, lover, and all-time favorite lab rat.

And to our grandchildren,
Emma, Eddie, Leo, Sophia, and Bodhi.
Alex and Gracie, too.
Eat well and thrive!

Contents

Foreword

Empowering Health

BY DAVID PERLMUTTER, M.D.

Are we merely the product of our genetic inheritance, or is our health destiny determined by the lifestyle and nutritional choices we make? This seemingly irreconcilable dichotomy has persisted at least dating back to the original description of DNA by James Watson and Francis Crick in 1953. In the years following their discovery, the pendulum of scientific opinion has swung back and forth, at times more supportive of the influence of genetic inheritance (nature) while at other times favoring the role of modifiable extrinsic factors (nurture) as playing the dominant role in determining health outcome.

In February 2001, Craig Venter and his colleagues published the results of their successful efforts to sequence the entire human genome. This landmark effort, appearing in the journal *Nature,* clearly influenced the nature-versus-nurture debate in favor of the former as the inner workings of the code of life were revealed, to the amazement of scientists and lay individuals alike.

For several years following Venter's remarkable publication, scientific sentiment remained fairly dedicated to the notion that much of what went on in terms of health, resistance to disease, and even longevity, were hardwired into our genetic code. And this mentality was supported, to some degree, by the ever-expanding body of knowledge in the area of DNA research.

In just the past several years, however, we are seeing a resurgence of scientific research that clearly supports the nurture side of the dichotomy, emphasizing the critical role of factors like nutrition, management of stress, sleep, and physical exercise in determining health outcome.

So what are we to believe? Are we truly merely the product of our inheritance, or does what appears on our breakfast plates matter most in terms of our health destiny?

In the pages that follow, Dr. Joan Borysenko masterfully brings resolution to this long-standing debate by revealing that nature and nurture are fully engaged in a dance. The empowering vanguard science of *epigenetics* reveals that the very choices we make in terms of what and how we eat, drink, smoke, love, or choose to avoid provide active and dynamic instructions to what was formerly considered an immutable set of instructions held in our DNA.

The PlantPlus Diet Solution provides a user-friendly, actionable plan designed to allow each of us the ability to implement the very latest scientific research to modify the expression of our genetic code for positive health results.

Further, Dr. Borysenko deftly explores the powerful influence upon human health of the *microbiome*, the more than 100 trillion bacteria living within each of us. And when you consider that each of us harbors more than 1,000 different species of bacteria in our microbiome, each species with its own unique genetic signature, the notion of positively influencing *their* genetic expression through lifestyle choices empowers us even further as we seek a long and healthy life.

The empowerment offered by *The PlantPlus Diet Solution* is thus about the tools you will receive to bring about life-sustaining changes in the expression of not only your genetic code, but also that of your microbiome. Lowering carbohydrates and avoiding grains while welcoming healthful fats back to the table have well-described direct physiological benefits. But when you embrace the strategic role of these and other sensible lifestyle changes revealed in this book in terms of their roles in augmenting positive gene expression, the potential health benefits are boundless.

Prologue

Dietary Genesis

In the beginning, God covered the earth with broccoli and cauliflower and spinach, green and yellow and red vegetables of all kinds, so Man and Woman would live long and healthy lives.

Then using God's bountiful gifts, Satan created ice cream and doughnuts. And Satan said, "You want hot fudge with that?" And Man said, "Yes!" And Woman said, "I'll have another with sprinkles." And lo, they gained ten pounds.

So God said, "Try my fresh green salad."

And Satan presented crumbled blue-cheese dressing and garlic toast on the side. And Man and Woman unfastened their belts following the repast.

God then said, "I have sent you heart-healthy vegetables and olive oil in which to lightly sauté the wholesome vegetables."

And Satan brought forth deep-fried coconut shrimp, chicken-fried steak so big it needed its own platter, and chocolate cheesecake for dessert. And Man's glucose levels spiked through the roof.

God then brought forth running shoes so that his Children might lose those extra pounds.

And Satan came forth with a cable TV with remote control so Man would not have to toil changing the channels. And Man and Woman laughed and cried before the flickering light and started wearing stretch jogging suits.

Then God brought forth lean meat so that Man might consume fewer calories and still satisfy his appetite.

And Satan created the 99-cent double cheeseburger, and said, "You want fries with that?" And Man replied, "Yes! And supersize 'em!" And Man went into cardiac arrest.

God sighed and created quadruple bypass surgery.

And Satan created HMOs.

— Clever Author Unknown

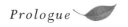

Dietary Re-Genesis

Thus unfolds the biblical saga of Dietary De-Generation up unto and including this very day.

The Earth and the Water, the Children and the Elders, have met the enemy.

And in accordance with the Sacred Prophecy of Pogo . . . Behold! The Enemy is Us.

That's the bad news.

But lo! It is also the good news.

What we tore down in the name of convenience and profit, we can rebuild in the name of goodness, taste, and sanity so that our children and our children's children may live long, healthy, creative, loving lives on a planet that can nourish us all.

— Joan Borysenko

Introduction

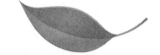

Confused About
What to Eat?

"Quod ali cibus est aliis fuat acre venenum."
("What is food for one man may be bitter poison to others.")

— LUCRETIUS, 1ST CENTURY B.C.

Most people I talk to are downright confused and frustrated about what to eat and why. Is whole grain the staff of life, or can it damage the brain or the gut? Is wheat a particularly scary bogeyman or not? Is eating an egg really as bad as smoking a cigarette? What about meat? Dairy? Fish? Soy? My intention is to give you the information you need to decide which of these foods (the *Plus* foods in the PlantPlus Diet Solution) are right for you.

Before I tell you who I am and why I've spent three years researching and writing this book, let me tell you who I'm not. I'm not a physician, nutritionist, or chef. I have no supplements to sell, nor any ax to grind. I'm a regular person who got a diagnosis of hypertension at about the same time my husband, Gordon, discovered that he had plaque in his arteries, putting him at risk for heart attack and stroke. We decided to see if changing our diet might help.

That was the beginning of several years of concentrated diet sleuthing. First we tried a low-fat, high-carb, mostly vegan diet. After 14 months of sticking resolutely to that heart-approved program, unfortunately, we continued to lose ground. My hypertension worsened, and while some of Gordon's cardiac indicators improved, others got worse. To add insult to injury, we both gained weight. While many other people, including President Bill Clinton, thrive on a high-carb, low-fat diet—and there is solid research to support it for people with heart disease—for us it wasn't the hoped-for panacea.

It was frustrating to try so hard, and to believe in a diet with such evangelistic fervor, only to lose ground. So, using my Harvard Medical School doctorate in cell biology to good advantage, I dove into the literature on nutrition and got better acquainted with some of the disastrous national policies that shaped our health, and our approach to heart disease, over the past half century.

Ever since President Dwight D. Eisenhower was diagnosed with heart disease in 1961 and put on a low-fat diet, lowering dietary fat while increasing carbohydrates became nutritional dogma in spite of some mighty sketchy research. Yes, the rates of heart disease have gone down, but the experts don't think that diet was involved. Less smoking, better emergency medicine, more long-term care, fewer cases of rheumatic fever, and healthier moms who bore higher-birth-weight babies are the likely causes of the decrease in heart disease over the past 60 years.

Ironically the very dietary changes that were put in place specifically to reduce the incidence of heart disease, which still claims the lives of one in four Americans, ignited an epidemic of obesity, diabetes, metabolic derangement, and Alzheimer's disease instead.

In 1960 the United States was 16th in life expectancy compared to 191 other countries worldwide. The most recent data I could find, for the year 2012, was published in *The World Factbook* compiled by the CIA. The United States ranked 51st in life expectancy, behind Bosnia and Herzegovina, barely nosing out Guam.

We're at a turning point where children now being born in the United States are the first generation whose life span is on track to be shorter than that of their parents. They are slated to live, on average, an alarmingly short 69 years. One single medical recommendation—to eat low-fat foods—spawned a high-carb feeding frenzy that may be the single most expensive mistake, in terms of both human suffering and economics, ever made in the name of evidence-based medicine.

Three things have to happen to reverse the health trends that are fast eroding both quality of life and our economy, both personally and as a nation:

1. **Minimize refined carbs.** It's time to call off our national love affair with what some nutritionists call "crap carbs," high-glycemic-index carbohydrates, devoid of fiber, which come from refined grains and sugar that send your blood glucose soaring. As you'll read about shortly, these carbs are a major culprit in the health epidemic. Even whole grains can turn into sugar more quickly than some people's metabolism can handle.

2. **Eat a *carb-reasonable amount* of low-glycemic-index good carbs—the kind found in high-fiber whole vegetables and fruits.** The most basic practical consideration that governs how to eat for your metabolic type is simple: Given the environment in which we live, does the combination of our genetics, our gut microbes, and the food we eat (plus other factors that have yet to be discovered) lead us to be (1) exquisitely insulin sensitive, (2) moderately insulin sensitive, or (3) insulin resistant? Simple blood tests can tell you. The more insulin resistant you are, the fewer carbs you can eat without deranging your metabolism and setting yourself up for chronic disease.

3. **Personalize your diet for your unique physiology.** Beyond eating a diet composed largely of vegetables and fruits, some people will thrive on whole grains and legumes. Other people less so. Some people can

eat gluten, whereas others cannot. Certain folks can eat more fats than others, and fats of differing composition. Some people do well with dairy, and others not so much. And while meat is what I call a *Plus* food for many of us, it's less suitable for others.

There Is No One-Size-Fits-All Diet

We all have three genomes: the one we inherit from mom and dad; our microbiome (the gut microbes and their genes); and our epigenome (the control panel of environmental change agents that turn our genes on and off). These three genomes form the backbone of the new science of personalized nutrition.

"Deciding between the Atkins Diet, Mediterranean diet or a traditional low-fat/high-carbohydrates diet?" That's the opener to an article in *The Jerusalem Post* that highlights a study performed at Ben-Gurion University. The article concludes that there is no one-size-fits-all diet; however, "those on the low-carb diet did the best at keeping the weight off. . . . But the differences in the results between the three diets' menus were less important than how much of their diet consisted of vegetables."[1]

In the original article the authors write: "Universal predictors of successful weight loss in the rapid weight loss phase across all diet strategies are increasing the weight of intake of vegetables and decreasing the weight of intake of sweets and cakes."[2]

A diet rich in vegetables and at least some fruit is good for almost everyone. But it doesn't have to be all we eat—and in many cases, shouldn't be. Whether you're one of the 0.5 percent of Americans who prefer to be vegans (no animal products, including dairy or eggs), the 3.2 percent who are vegetarians (dairy and eggs but no animal flesh), or a member of the Great Omnivorous Majority, a diet based on whole, unprocessed foods with lots of nutrient-rich, calorie-sparse vegetables is a good starting point.

Until very recently there was no reliable way to know what your unique dietary needs were. Various writers suggested that your blood type or how fast you oxidized fats could be used to choose foods that were right for your body type, but those ideas haven't stood the test of time.

Consider this fact: When people are randomly assigned to specific diet types that vary in the amounts of carbs, fat, and protein, some people lose a lot of weight. Others lose little or none, and a few even gain weight. The factors that create so much variation compose the promising new field of personalized nutrition.

Christopher Gardner, Ph.D., director of nutrition studies at the Stanford Prevention Research Center and associate professor of medicine at Stanford University, carried out a couple of landmark studies that shed light on which people will lose the most weight on diets that vary in carb and fat content. His data suggests that insulin-resistant people lose more weight on a low-carb diet, while people who aren't insulin resistant do just as well on any of the major weight-loss diets.

In an interview in the *Nutrition Action Healthletter,* Gardner was asked if the big losers in his famous A to Z (Atkins to Zone) study, which we'll look at a little later, lost more weight because they adhered to their diets more closely. His response was, "Possibly. We think some people have a harder time adhering to a diet because it's the wrong one for them metabolically."[3]

In **Part I** of this book, I'll distill the scientific research you need to understand the fascinating world of metabolism and diet into tasty, digestible tidbits. I call these fun excursions into the world of scientific and nutritional literacy *Science Bites.* There's a lot to the science of food and metabolism, so feel free to skip around through these. You can think of them as a reference that you can go back to when you need to look something up.

Most of us do better at anything if we know exactly why we're doing it and what to expect. That's the point of the Science Bites. You'll understand the all-important connection between carbs, insulin, and fat storage. And it will make perfect sense why (if you're overweight) willpower alone won't help you, but eating a delicious PlantPlus Diet will—without ever restricting calories or going hungry.

When I give seminars on the PlantPlus way of life, most participants are delighted when their own inner scientist wakes up. How do you tell if you're carb resistant or carb sensitive? Why is it important to eat healthy fats? Why are some fats unhealthy? How do we tell which scientific studies are good and which are faulty? My hope is that this information will empower you to take charge of your health.

In **Part II**, I put on my psychologist's hat (I'm a licensed clinical psychologist as well as a scientist, and cofounder of one of the first mind-body clinics in the country). I'll help you create a relationship to food that's rewarding, healing, simple, and super satisfying. I was originally planning to call this book "The Plant-Plus Diet," but that was too limited in scope.

Changing your diet is about more than a brief stint of deprivation in the name of getting back into your skinny jeans. And you'd better take some photos if that day ever comes, since 95 percent of people who lose weight regain it within a year, often with "interest." What we need are fewer temporary weight-loss diets and more emphasis on learning how to create a healthy, enjoyable food lifestyle that's delicious and simple to maintain, especially given how busy most of us are. As a clinical psychologist, I'm going to tell you exactly how to do that.

It's interesting that the word *diet* itself actually comes from the Greek *diaita*, which means "a way of life." If you're willing to experiment with a PlantPlus way of life, you'll naturally optimize the function of your cells, tissues, and organs. Your weight will adjust to its natural balance point without any hunger or deprivation. And in many cases, you'll be able to reverse or improve chronic health problems ranging from diabetes to hypertension, from obesity to metabolic syndrome.

When I was doing the research for this book, it amazed me that few other books on diet had any information on how to outwit the cravings that are the death knell of most diets. Here you'll learn how to use mindfulness, cognitive, and breathing techniques to rewire your brain, reduce cravings, and enhance pleasure not only from food, but also from this entire miraculous life.

In **Part III**, we'll get down to business. I'll lay out a 28-Day Reboot for you. In these four weeks you'll have plenty to eat. I promise not only that you won't go hungry, but also that you'll enjoy some of the best food you've ever eaten. When the 28 days are over, based on both a simple battery of medical tests plus a self-test called the Medical Symptom Checklist that I've included for you in the Appendix (you'll fill this out both before and after the Reboot), you—or you and your physician—can review your health measures and see what your progress is like. In the Personalization phase, you can add back some of what's been eliminated in the Reboot, one food at a time. This may be grains, beans, or red meat, for example. You'll track your responses to these foods both in the short run and over a longer period.

In **Part IV**, finally, it's time to eat! First we'll look at a list of my favorite Superfoods (Dr. Joan's Superfoods) so that when we get to the recipes, you'll understand why I've included them. There's also a chapter on eating well for less, and instructions on eating PlantPlus *Lite* if you want a dietary change but aren't ready for the whole journey of Reboot and Personalization.

Thanks for reading with an open mind and a willing heart. The time to change our national and personal way of eating has come. Peter Attia, M.D., a former health-care consultant for McKinsey & Company, wrote on his website The Eating Academy: "The U.S. spends over **$2.7 trillion** per year on healthcare—nearly **19% of our GDP,** and more than any other country. Even if no other aspect of our spending increases in the next 20 years, the cost of healthcare alone will bankrupt us as a country."

Why Is the PlantPlus Diet a Solution?

What's true for us in terms of our personal health and the health of our economy is also true for our planet. It's in crisis. I'm not an alarmist, but it's ostrich-like to dispute the facts. Earth truly is at a tipping point. Global warming, increasing pollution,

The PlantPlus Diet Solution

and agricultural practices that deplete the soil, poison the water, and kill our beneficial bacterial allies (and eventually us) are hard to ignore. What we do to the Earth, we do to ourselves. Our elders, who are succumbing to an epidemic of Alzheimer's disease, are like canaries in the mine. So are the increased number of autistic children. Are you overweight? Diabetic? Depressed? Anxious? You're a canary in the mine as well.

Something has gone terribly wrong with our national health and well-being, and it's high time for the tide to turn. The PlantPlus Diet—a scientific, metabolically personalized, whole-foods approach to health—is also a *solution* to some of these pressing problems. If we as consumers refuse to eat junk foods, genetically modified foods, pesticide-riddled produce, and products made from factory-farmed animals, we'll be healthier and so will our precious children. Furthermore, eating the PlantPlus way—personalized for your own unique metabolism—is empowering. It's a step you can take to ensure that you, your children, your children's children, and the Earth herself endure and prosper for the good of us all.

Author's Note

This book is meant solely as an educational tool and should not be construed as medical advice. Please check with your physician before beginning any dietary regime. Hopefully you have, or will find, a physician who is willing to be your partner in discovery; who can make sure that any dietary changes you make are consistent with your physical condition and any medications you might be taking; who can order and interpret the appropriate tests to help personalize your diet for your unique physiology; and who can adjust any medications you might be taking as needed. The information in this book is not meant to replace, override, or contradict the advice of your physician. Both the author and the publisher disclaim any liability in connection with the use of this book.

xxvi

PART I

SCIENCE BITES

The Science Bites to come are meant to help you understand why the Standard American Diet (SAD) is gradually killing us off, what metabolism is all about, why the body needs certain nutrients, how to get smart when it comes to interpreting studies, why being fat makes you hungry and how to beat it, what the diet studies reveal, how your three sets of genetic modulators regulate what diet is best for you, how to calculate a carb-reasonable diet, what medical tests to ask for, and what you really need to know to personalize your own diet.

But before you start reading the Science Bites, please go to the Appendix, make a couple of copies of the Medical Symptom Checklist, and fill one out now. Put it in a safe place since it will give you a health baseline for comparison. You probably know enough to begin *PlantPlus Lite:* eat plenty of vegetables and a few fruits a day, and eliminate all grain flour (not just wheat and gluten-containing flour, but all flour and baked goods, gluten-free or not) and sugar from all sources, including agave nectar, honey, and high-fructose corn syrup.

If you gradually move in the PlantPlus Lite direction while learning about the finer points of what to eat and why, and how to personalize your diet further, you'll be on your way to a better mood and better health.

So let's get going!

CHAPTER 1

What's Up, Doc?

"One cannot think well, love well, sleep well,
if one has not dined well."

— VIRGINIA WOOLF, *A ROOM OF ONE'S OWN*

Tired, cranky, got headaches, bellyaches, or belly fat? How about diabetes, high blood pressure, or coronary artery disease? Got an autoimmune condition, an allergy, an immune deficiency, or an inflammatory condition like arthritis? Depressed, anxious, addicted, or having trouble sleeping? Overweight, obese, or just plain bloated? How about dementia, Alzheimer's disease, or cancer?

These chronic illnesses and mood disorders, all of which have some association with metabolic problems due to poor diet, are endemic to our society.

It's estimated that 25 to 30 percent of the population is now insulin resistant (prediabetic) because of the carb-rich foods that form the backbone of the Standard American Diet (SAD). Add in the toxins we ingest—a result of pesticides, herbicides, GMOs, food additives, and the consumption of oxidized vegetable oils rich in omega-6 fatty acids—and you get the perfect storm. When even health-conscious folks like my husband, Gordon, and I fall prey to the epidemic of chronic disease, it's clear that we need to become better educated as a society before we become extinct.

The Girth of the Nation

Almost 70 percent of American adults are overweight. It's no wonder that Europeans are often shocked when they come to the U.S. and see how much fatter we are compared to the citizens of European Union nations, many of which—like Italy and France—are known for their rich, delicious cuisine.

Over a third of Americans are now more than just a tad overweight. Forget about losing those stubborn five or ten pounds. How about those 20, 30, 40, 50, or 100 pounds? Think I'm exaggerating? One in 20 American adults is indeed extremely obese—100 pounds or more over their optimal weight. Our kids aren't faring much better. A *third* of them are overweight. Of those, nearly one in five are officially obese with a BMI (body mass index) of 30 or more. Take a moment to imagine that. . . .

Or perhaps you see the problem up close and personal in your own children, grandchildren, or their classmates. When I went to grade school and high school in the 1950s and early 1960s, an overweight kid was a rarity. Most everyone was thin. Most of what we ate were whole foods, since the processed-food industry was just gearing up for a hostile takeover of the American palate and pocketbook.

My mom, who once made everything we ate from scratch, became smitten with Pop-Tarts when I was an adolescent. Those processed breakfast pastries were a harbinger of things to come. The unholy alliance between Bad Science, which blamed fat for heart disease, and Big Food launched half a century of low-fat, high-carb cardio-mania that made our country the fattest country in the world until Mexico nosed (or butted) us out of top place in 2013.

Fit but Still Fat?

I used to think that overweight people just ate too much and exercised too little. But that's not always true. Many overweight or obese people do exercise, and they may also eat what most of us would consider a healthy diet, and not too much of it.

So what gives?

Books on diet and nutrition sometimes ponder just this question, citing cases of people who are fit but still fat. The wife of cardiologist William Davis, M.D., author of the best-selling book *Wheat Belly,* is a triathlete and trainer of triathletes. Dr. Davis observed that about a third of these elite athletes are overweight. While exercise is one of the best things you can do for health and mood overall, the truth is that it has very little to do with weight.

C'mon now. Do you really plan on running for half an hour to burn off the calories in a single cookie?

Groundbreaking health journalist Gary Taubes, author of *Good Calories, Bad Calories* and *Why We Get Fat,* may have at least part of the answer for how it's possible to be fit (at least in terms of exercise tolerance) but fat . . . or simply fat even though you don't necessarily overeat. On the basis of a meticulous (and once controversial) five-year project researching and vetting studies on which the high-carb, low-fat dietary dogma is based, Taubes concluded that *obesity is a fat accumulation disorder rather than an eating disorder.*

That's a very interesting hypothesis, so let me repeat it. If Taubes is correct—and progressively more scientists and physicians are adopting his point of view—then *the obesity problem isn't just about eating too many calories. It's about the physiological effect of the foods we've been encouraged to eat—namely carbs—on our hormones.*

The hormone insulin in particular.

When we eat and blood sugar increases, insulin shuttles glucose out of the bloodstream into cells where it's either burned for energy or stored as glycogen—a starchy polymer of glucose—or fat. Taubes explains the effects of insulin this way:

First, when insulin levels are elevated, we accumulate fat in our fat tissue; when these levels fall, we liberate fat from the fat tissue and burn it for fuel. This has been known since the early 1960s and has never been controversial. Second, our insulin levels are effectively determined by the carbohydrates we eat. . . . 'Carbohydrate is driving insulin is driving fat,' is how George Cahill, a former professor of medicine at Harvard Medical School, recently described this to me.[1]

Eating carbs high in the *glycemic index* (GI) results in the liberation of glucose into the bloodstream. The higher the GI of a food, the faster it's metabolized into sugar. The more sugar you eat, the more fat you store. That's why eating low-GI carbs helps you stay trim.

But sugar aside, there's another reason why eating too many "crap carbs" (the high-GI kind found in processed foods) makes us fat. The lack of fiber and nutrients in these foods lays the groundwork for what microbiologists call *dysbiosis,* a disturbance in the community of our all-important gut microbes. Our *probiotics*—the friendly gut microbes that you'll learn about in Chapter 14—need to eat *prebiotics*—fiber-rich whole foods—in order to flourish and fight off bad bacteria, protect our gut lining, synthesize vitamins and neurotransmitters, and help us absorb nutrients from the foods we eat.

Carbs and Diabetes

All the elements that combined to create the perfect storm of chronic disease culminated in a tsunami that pediatric endocrinologist Francine Kaufman, M.D., dubbed *diabesity,* obesity accompanied by type 2 diabetes.

Diabesity has already reached epidemic proportions in both children and adults and continues to increase at an alarming rate.

As of 2012, diabetes was already a $245 billion business, up from $174 billion in 2007. $176 billion went for direct medical costs. Another $69 billion went for indirect costs (disability and work loss). All told, the average medical expenditures for people with diagnosed diabetes (it's estimated that another 7 million people have undiagnosed diabetes) were 2.3 times higher than for people without the illness.[2]

In fact, 8.3 percent of the U.S. population—25.8 million children and adults—have diabetes. Another 79 million people have prediabetes, the insulin resistance and metabolic syndrome that lead to diabetes. The good news is that metabolic syndrome and prediabetes can often be reversed—and quickly—by a low-glycemic, nutritionally personalized PlantPlus Diet.

And what about the epidemic of Alzheimer's disease? One in three seniors has evidence of dementia at the time of death. *Furthermore, the incidence of Alzheimer's has increased 70 percent between 2000 and 2010.* There's evidence that nutrition (or lack of) is a powerful risk factor for this dreaded disease. Just as I was putting the finishing touches on the manuscript for this book, *Grain Brain* by neurologist David Perlmutter, M.D., who kindly wrote the Foreword for this book, hit multiple bestseller lists. We cover much the same scientific database, but if you have a specific interest in neurogenerative diseases and Alzheimer's, Perlmutter's book is a bonanza of information.

But even if you're not interested in overt neurological conditions, all of us want to be mentally sharp. We also want to avoid the Scylla and Charybdis of anxiety and depression. The bottom line is that eating a diet high in carbs decreases BDNF—*brain-derived neurotrophic factor,* a hormone that maintains neurons, encourages their growth, and enables the brain to repair and remodel itself.

Now that you have an overview of some of the health problems we face as a nation, in the next chapter we'll get more specific about how some of the common foods we eat create a disease-causing environment in the body. There are five major food-related problems that a PlantPlus lifestyle is meant to correct. Read on and discover what I call the Five Pillars of Dietary Doom.

CHAPTER 2

The Five Pillars of Dietary Doom

"I come from a home where gravy is a beverage."

— ERMA BOMBECK

If you're interested in nutrition, you've probably read a lot about why the Standard American Diet (SAD) is killing us off. But a lot of what passes for nutritional information comes down to generalities or turns out to be bad science, outmoded theory, snake oil, or unfounded opinion. This is all so confusing that most people I know, clever and well-meaning though they are, throw up their hands in despair and end up ignoring the hidden culprits in the kitchen.

In the spirit of nutritional literacy, this chapter gets to the root of the processes whereby what we eat might simultaneously be eating us. Remember, the most important dietary changes you can make are:

1. Banish fake foods from your life.

2. Welcome whole foods—mostly vegetables and fruits.

3. Banish bad fats and substitute good fats.

4. Find your unique Plus Foods.

5. Let what you eat delight your senses. No one willingly gives up the foods they love for something that tastes worse. Make no mistake. Eating delicious food that nourishes your body and soul is an upgrade, not a medieval hair shirt designed for doing penance.

In this Science Bite, I'll explain why some foods need to be banished from your life because they lay the foundation for dietary doom: (1) oxidative stress; (2) inflammation; (3) glycation; (4) micronutrient insufficiency; and (5) dysbiosis caused by fiber insufficiency and antibiotics. Later on you'll learn about the good foods in a PlantPlus lifestyle that help reverse the effects of the Standard American Diet.

Before you groan, cheer up. This is interesting stuff, so take a deep breath and open yourself up to a new world of foodie fun. You'll enjoy your PlantPlus lifestyle even more when you know what it's doing—and undoing—for you.

Pillar #1: Oxidative Stress

All the chronic degenerative diseases that are so rampant today—including diabetes, hypertension, atherosclerosis, heart failure, arthritis, cancer, neurodegenerative disorders, and other conditions associated with premature aging—are linked to oxidative stress. But chances are you don't actually know what oxidation is, other than it's not such a good thing.

Oxidation is a natural biochemical process that occurs all the time in your body. The oxygen that provides energy for life exists in the form of O_2—two atoms of oxygen bonded into a single molecule. During metabolism, atoms of the O_2 molecule can lose an electron. The electron-deficient oxygen is then incorporated into a variety of molecules called Reactive Oxygen Species (ROS). ROS, known as *free radicals*, have a natural function in cell-to-cell signaling and communication. But here's the rub. Normal oxidation can easily ramp up into *oxidative stress*.

Here's what happens. Free radicals are created by pesticides and herbicides used to grow produce, the excess carbohydrates in both refined and whole foods, overexposure to sunlight, and other sources of pollution in the environment, including electromagnetic frequencies.

These free radicals then go on a spree. They steal electrons from other molecules throughout the body. The resultant oxidation (loss of an electron to oxygen) damages proteins, lipids (fats), and DNA. Let me give you an example that you're familiar with. When iron oxidizes, the result is rust. Just as rust can age your tailpipe, oxidation also ages your body.

Atherosclerosis, or hardening of the arteries, is not actually due to LDL-C or total "bad" cholesterol levels per se. In fact, about half of all people who have heart attacks have normal cholesterol levels. Cholesterol-containing plaque develops because of the damage inflicted on arterial walls through *oxidized* small LDL particles and perhaps oxidized HDL (the good cholesterol) as well. The rogue oxidized molecules initiate a cascade of harmful immune reactions that result in cholesterol being deposited in the artery walls.

Oxidized cholesterol has long been recognized as a villain in the atherosclerotic process, although it's the rare physician who will tell you about it because most physicians aren't aware of the research. Ironically, the low-fat, high-carb diet recommended to prevent or even reverse atherosclerosis can—for some people— actually add to the oxidative stress that's causing the problem to begin with.

Amino acids that form proteins are also prone to oxidation by free radicals. Oxidized amino acids change the way proteins fold, which in turn changes their function. For a protein, form follows function. Keeping the correct shape is a nonnegotiable necessity. Think about a child's Lego blocks. If you leave them on a radiator and the blocks melt and lose their shape even a little, they can no longer effectively lock on to one another. The result is that they lose some or all of their function. Then, of course, someone has to clean up the mess. In the body, that's called detoxification.

> Oxidative stress becomes a problem when there are more ROS (free radicals) than the body is able to detoxify. Here is where a PlantPlus Diet shines because it is rich in naturally occurring antioxidants.

Antioxidants

Antioxidants are substances that quench (satisfy) free radicals by donating an electron to them. The body makes its own antioxidants, thankfully, but in most cases not enough to neutralize the extra ROS. Plants, however, have an innate antioxidant system to protect themselves from oxidative stresses brought on by drought, ultraviolet radiation, temperature extremes, and the like. So eating an antioxidant-rich PlantPlus Diet plentiful in greens and colored fruits and vegetables not only helps quench free radicals but also has an effect on how your body manufactures its own antioxidants.

Colorful vegetables and fruits are known for their antioxidant and antioxidant-stimulating properties. These are due to the activity of phytochemicals called *flavonoids*, or plant pigments, a word that comes from the Latin for "yellow." A large scientific literature documents not only the antioxidant effects of flavonoids but also their antiviral, anti-allergen, anti-inflammatory, and anticancer properties. Flavonoids are the reason why you've been told to eat a rainbow of colors each day (red, orange, yellow, green, blue, and purple). In Part IV, the recipe section, you'll discover simple, delicious, carb-reasonable ways to do that.

Fortunately for the PlantPlus lifestyle, some not-so-colorful plant products are also rich in flavonoids. Black tea, green tea, white tea, and dark chocolate are exceptionally concentrated sources of flavonoids, as is coffee—the single-most widely used antioxidant in the United States. Years of trying to indict coffee as a health threat has finally come to an end as long as you can tolerate and break down caffeine easily so that you don't become anxious and jittery.

When we take a look at the emerging field of genetic testing in a later Science Bite, and consider what it can and can't do to help you personalize your nutrition, you'll discover that one of the genes that can be tested for involves the efficiency with which a person metabolizes caffeine. I'm a fast metabolizer and love to start the day with a homemade cappuccino. As a devoted coffee maven, I'd turn to decaf if I were a slow caffeine metabolizer. But all decaf is not created equal. Most commercial brands use poisonous solvents to leach out the caffeine. Residues of these solvents can add to oxidative stress. Look for water-processed decaf. That gives you antioxidants without any oxidizing solvent residues.

Now that you know what oxidative stress is, and why plants are so important in reducing it, the next obvious question is: Why do so many people discount—and even make fun of—organic produce?

Why Organic?

When a 2012 study out of Stanford University[1] reported no significant nutritional differences between organic and commercially grown produce, a lot of folks felt vindicated in their choice of cheaper nonorganic foods. But the problem lies not in what the study found—that the organic and nonorganic produce tested had similar nutrient profiles. The real problem with conventionally grown produce is the pesticides and weed killers used in their production, which create oxidative stress.

In Part IV, you'll read about the Environmental Working Group's "Dirty Dozen Plus" and "Clean Fifteen" produce categories. Buying dirty produce (intensely sprayed crops like apples, strawberries, and kale) isn't such a good idea. Organic is a much better choice. But if you're buying asparagus, sweet potatoes, or cantaloupe, for example, it's less important to think organic—at least in terms of pesticide residues.

Pillar #2: Inflammation

Agricultural chemical pollution isn't the only source of oxidative stress. Most commercially processed foods are loaded with other chemicals. These may include dyes, preservatives, emulsifiers, flavorings, and a whole host of chemicals that stabilize, texturize, deodorize, and—to my thinking—metaphorically plasticize these products to extend their shelf life. Some of these chemicals can lead to an immune reaction called *inflammation*.

> The word *inflammation* comes from the Latin *inflammatio*, "to set on fire." We hear a lot about inflammation these days, since rigorous research has clearly established it as the final common pathway in the development of almost all chronic diseases, as well as in the frailty that accompanies aging.

There are two types of inflammation: acute and chronic. Acute inflammation is a normal and necessary immunological response. If you get a splinter, for example, acute inflammation fights off potential infection and helps bring the foreign object to the skin surface where it can be expelled. The area around the splinter gets red, hot, and swollen as immune cells flood in to kill invading bacteria, viruses, fungi, or parasites. Following the cellular battle, another crew of immune cells arrives on the scene to clean up the mess and haul off the dead bodies for recycling. Then everyone goes home and calls it a day. That's good inflammation.

Bad or chronic inflammation, on the other hand, doesn't simply resolve itself and go away. Immune cells keep on trying to protect the body from threat. The problem lies in the fact that there *is* no immediate invasion calling the immune troops into action. Instead, immune cells stay triggered by oxidized proteins and fats and by immune factors called *pro-inflammatory cytokines* made both by belly fat and as a response to physical and emotional stress.

Belly fat, as we'll check out more closely in a later Science Bite, is more than unsightly flab under the skin. It's visceral fat, which accumulates *between* your internal organs. This special kind of fat functions as a gland that releases hormones as well as inflammatory immune factors.

A 2012 article in *Medical News Today* discussed research performed at the Fred Hutchinson Cancer Research Center in Seattle, Washington. Postmenopausal obese or overweight women who lost at least 5 percent of their body weight had significant drops in inflammation levels. That's very good news. The reporter quoted lead author Anne McTiernan, M.D., Ph.D., as saying, "Both obesity and inflammation have been shown to be related to several types of cancer, and this study shows that if you reduce weight, you can reduce inflammation as well."[2]

To lose weight, we need to lose the excess carbs that show up as *glycation,* the third Pillar of Dietary Doom. Glycation in turn fuels the fire of inflammation in a vicious and deadly cycle.

Pillar #3: Glycation

Glycation is a chemical reaction that occurs when a sugar molecule binds to a protein or a lipid. The root of the word comes from *glykýs,* the Greek word for "sweet." Hyperglycemia, for example, means that your blood is too sweet—you've got more glucose on board than your body can process.

Excess glucose creates a sticky carbohydrate sludge referred to as *advanced glycation end products (AGEs).* This sludge creates oxidative stress and inflammation, which as I've just mentioned is the root cause of all degenerative diseases. Why does that matter?

Advanced glycation end products can and do age us prematurely. The more AGEs accumulate, the more chronic conditions associated with aging appear even in the young. For example, nondiabetic children fed a typical American diet high in refined carbs can develop plaque in their arteries by the time they are two years old.[3]

Now think on this: *AGEs stay with you and continue to accumulate for your entire life, since the body has no way to excrete them.* They get into your tissues and stiffen them, getting in the way of proper function. Hypertension is related to the deposition of AGEs in the wall of blood vessels,[4] as is heart failure. While both heart attacks and cardiac damage are more prevalent in people with diabetes, any person who eats more carbs than his or her body can handle is at risk for developing cardiac problems.

AGEs are also deposited in the brain, where they're implicated in neurological conditions that range from mild cognitive impairment to Alzheimer's and Parkinson's disease. Scientists are trying to find ways to dislodge AGEs from our tissues, but so far they haven't had much luck.

Whoa. Wait just a minute here.

What does it mean that we have no innate mechanism to move AGE sludge out of our body?

The body is too smart to have evolved with such a fatal flaw. It's more reasonable to assume that we didn't evolve to eat a diet rich in sweets because they weren't widely available in ancestral times. Honey was once a scarce commodity as was fruit, which was seasonal and sour. Likewise, grain, which our body breaks down into sugar, wasn't available before our Neolithic ancestors learned to cultivate it about 10,000 years ago, as the Paleo diet

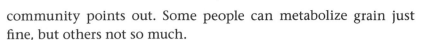

community points out. Some people can metabolize grain just fine, but others not so much.

Glucose on the loose, a result of eating more carbs that you can immediately process, results in blood sugar spikes. Each one of us has a differing ability to keep glucose where it belongs, inside our cells where it generates energy, as we'll cover in more detail in the Science Bites on insulin and insulin resistance.

An important part of personalizing your diet concerns monitoring your medical symptoms, weight, and medical tests to find out how many carbs *you* can eat without overwhelming your body's ability to keep glucose inside your cells where it generates energy instead of accumulating as AGEs.

Perhaps the main reason why AGEs age us, whether we have diabetes or not, is because they're inflammatory. Think on that and perhaps it will help you put on the brakes when you're tempted to buy a six-pack of cupcakes or sodas, a box of cookies, a package of bagels, or a pizza. None of these foods is going to kill you outright or even overnight. They're okay once in a while, but don't delude yourself into thinking that they're safe to eat habitually.

Pillar #4: Micronutrient Insufficiency

We may be a nation that's overweight, but the irony is that we're also undernourished. The calories provided by refined sugar are called empty because there are no micronutrients—vitamins, minerals, enzymes, or phytochemicals—in it. In other words, it has no nutritional value.

Whole plants, in contrast to refined foods high in carbs, contain as many as 10,000 different molecules referred to as *phytonutrients*. The flavonoid pigments that make berries red or purple are examples of phytonutrients. They're indispensable to millions of cellular reactions, yet we've just begun to scratch the surface in understanding them.

When we eat a diet of processed foods as opposed to fresh whole foods, critical micronutrients and phytonutrients go missing. For example, carotenoids are a family of about 600 different molecules found in carrots and other bright-orange and red plants like tomatoes and oranges, as well as in parsley and spinach. Some of the carotenoid molecules are antioxidants that stop fats from being oxidized and turned rancid by free radicals. Other carotenoids are precursors to vitamin A, modifiers of the immune response, and protectors against UV radiation, to name just a few other critical functions.

Physician Joel Fuhrman, M.D., is a champion of nutrient density. His simple "health equation" is H=N/C. *H* stands for your health. *N/C* stands for nutrient density per calorie. If you eat a nutrient-rich diet naturally high in fiber and low in calories, of course you'll lose weight. A high-fiber diet also favors the growth of gut microbes associated with being lean. A lack of fiber favors microbes associated with gaining weight. Furthermore, food has epigenetic effects. What you eat turns on and off different genes, including genes that protect against or predispose you to cancer.

Fuhrman is a staunch believer that low-fat diets are *not* the way to go, but he discourages the use of both olive oil and animal fats, concentrating on the fats naturally present in nuts, seeds, and avocados.

The PlantPlus Diet, in contrast, makes liberal use of olive oil, avocados, nuts and seeds, coconut oil, and organic dairy from pasture-grazed cows, sheep, and goats. These are *Plus* foods for many omnivores. Remember that the basis of a PlantPlus Diet *is still plants*. The Plus foods are additions, not the main course.

Pillar #5: Dysbiosis

Dysbiosis means a disturbance in the composition of your gut bacteria. You'll be learning a lot about gut bacteria in Science Bites to come. I'm completely captivated by this new field—arguably the most important scientific discovery since the human genome was mapped. Hundreds of studies about gut microbes are published every month. It's a real game changer in the field of health and nutrition as well as in the field of psychiatry since dysbiosis is related to anxiety, depression, and lack of stress hardiness.

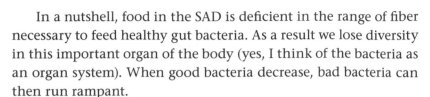

In a nutshell, food in the SAD is deficient in the range of fiber necessary to feed healthy gut bacteria. As a result we lose diversity in this important organ of the body (yes, I think of the bacteria as an organ system). When good bacteria decrease, bad bacteria can then run rampant.

Here's a short overview. We'll get into more detail shortly.

Geneticists are tracing human origins back to hunter-gatherer tribes in Africa. One such tribe, the Hadza, still lives a hunter-gatherer lifestyle in Tanzania. They live outside in nature and forage for their food. Although there's high infant mortality, the Hadza who make it through childhood live into their 60s, 70s, and 80s. They eat a lot of carbs in the form of dozens of different types of fibrous tubers that they dig for with long sticks. They also eat animals—from impala to wildebeest—that gather around watering holes in the dry season.

When the Hadza butcher the animals, which they eat in their entirety from head to tail, they wash the blood off their hands using the stomach contents of the animals—plant fiber. The point here is not to gross you out. The reason why I'm telling you this is to illustrate the fact that hunter-gathering people live outdoors in very close connection to a large variety of bacteria. Most Americans, on the other hand—unless they live on farms with animal neighbors—live in nearly hermetically sealed sterile environments.

But aren't bacteria bad?, you might be thinking. Well, some of them are. But many more of them are our allies. In fact, they are us! Microbes form an integral part of the human body. You and I are made up of a community of microbial and mammalian cells that are part of a symbiotic *supraorganism.*[5] Your "primitive" bacterial cells outnumber your eukaryotic (nucleated) cells by approximately ten to one. Whereas your mammalian cells have only about *23,000 genes*, your 100 trillion microorganisms contain about *3,000,000 genes*.

The various types of flora that make up our microbiome (the community of bacteria that reside in the body and their genes) are the first line of defense against pathogens from the outside world. They're like temple guards surrounding the entire body, both inside and out. The integrity of your microbiome is therefore paramount to your health. And unlike the Hadza, our bacterial community is no longer diverse and robust. It's gotten puny with overgrowths of bacterial species that cause obesity, food poisoning, and life-threatening infections like *Clostridium difficile,* or *C. diff.*

For our immediate purposes, we'll focus on the bacteria that live in our colon. While we think of the gut as inside the body, technically speaking it's also outside, contiguous with the epidermis or skin at both ends. The process of digestion extracts nutrients from food. Through elegant mechanisms that we'll touch upon shortly, bacteria aid nutrient absorption so that the body can grow itself, renew itself, make repairs, and have the fuel it needs to function.

When I taught microscopic anatomy to students at the Tufts University School of Medicine early in my career, they were fascinated by the fact that mitochondria—the energy plants within our cells—are derived from bacteria that took up residence in eukaryotic cells one to two billion years ago. These microscopic invaders learned to generate adenosine triphosphate (ATP), the currency of cellular energy, from glucose.

That energy-producing symbiosis allowed single-nucleated cells to join into multicellular, cooperative colonies. Cells within those colonies then specialized for the purpose of what some scientists call the Three F's: feeding, fighting, and, well, to be polite here, mating—the basic necessities for survival. Glucose was the fuel for this stunning evolutionary diversification. The result was a progression from single-celled organisms to multicellular organisms, and over the millennia to vertebrates like us.

Justin Sonnenburg, Ph.D., a microbiologist at Stanford, has an interesting take on the human relationship to our bacterial partners. He suggests that human beings are "an elaborate vessel optimized for the growth and spread of our microbial inhabitants." That's a humbling thought.

Sonnenburg's take on things reminds me of Lewis Thomas, M.D., whose science essays published as *The Lives of a Cell: Notes of a Biology Watcher* and *The Medusa and the Snail* captivated the

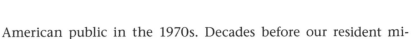
American public in the 1970s. Decades before our resident microbes were a serious subject of study, Thomas wrote:

> My mitochondria comprise a very large proportion of me. I cannot do the calculation, but I suppose there is almost as much of them in sheer dry bulk as there is the rest of me. Looked at in this way, I could be taken for a very large, motile colony of respiring bacteria, operating a complex system of nuclei, microtubules, and neurons for the pleasure and sustenance of their families, and running, at the moment, a typewriter.[6]

Most of the 100 trillion members of our microbiome are helpful little beasties like the ones that evolved into mitochondria. They have jobs that range from blocking harmful bacteria like salmonella or certain species of *E. coli* from invading our body, to helping in the prevention of type 1 diabetes in children, to extracting nutrients from the food we ingest, to manufacturing neurotransmitters that allow us to adapt to our environment and regulate our mood, to guiding our evolution and physiology.

A few of the microbes can in some instances be pathogenic, like the *Helicobacter pylori* that cause stomach ulcers; strains of *E. coli* that are life-threatening; and other strains that produce no symptoms at all, except indirectly in people with Crohn's disease. Those folks, perhaps because of a preexisting genetic susceptibility, mount an excessive immune response to the *E. coli*, generating a powerful inflammatory environment that creates pain, malabsorption, diarrhea, and ulcerations.

Gut bacteria manufacture a host of products critical to our health like vitamins and short-chain fatty acids; they are an integral part of our immune system—80 percent of which is located in our gut; and they affect the way that we develop in the womb and how our organs function.[7]

It's clear that what we know about our bacterial allies is far less than what remains to be discovered. And mark my words: The little we know about nutrition now will burgeon in the next few years, radically revising a lot of old information about conditions that range from neurological problems to heart disease, and from diabetes to obesity.

I'm happy to say that we're on the cusp of a dietary revolution. For that reason some of what you read here might have been rendered obsolete by the time this book is published. And no, that doesn't make me feel bad. If you read this book through, you'll become an educated eater more capable of vetting the research, as well as the nonscientific anecdotal claims that bombard us constantly with eat this, not that, or that, or that.

Now that you know about the Five Pillars of Dietary Doom (a little melodrama is helpful at times), let's take a look at what we eat in terms of macronutrient composition: the role fats, carbs, and proteins play in our metabolism.

CHAPTER 3

The Three Macronutrients:

Proteins, Fats, and Carbs

"Human beings do not eat nutrients; they eat food."

— Mary Catherine Bateson

When my youngest son, Andrei, was seven or eight, he was delighted with his newfound knowledge of the four major food groups gleaned from his second-grade school buddies. They were, he told me with a giggle, cookies, pies, candy, and cakes. Since those items were in short supply around our house, Andrei considered his four fantasy food groups not only entertaining but also possibly instructive for his dorky mom who packed healthy lunches that no one wanted to trade him for.

In this little Science Bite, we'll take a quick look at the three real macronutrients that make up the food we eat: *fats, carbohydrates*, and *proteins*. Knowing how your body turns these nutrients into fuel and building materials for cells, tissues, and organs will help you understand the perennial controversy about how much of each macronutrient is needed for good health. Since all the major diets that we'll look at in later chapters espouse different percentages of macronutrients, it's important to know a little bit about them. It's also good to bear in mind that:

1. There's no magic macronutrient formula that works for every body.

2. The only macronutrient not essential for life is carbohydrate.

3. There are good fats and bad fats.

4. Protein is the ultimate skinny food because it takes so much energy to digest.

A Brief Food-as-Fuel Overview

Carbohydrates are molecules of sugar, starch, or cellulose that are broken down into simple sugars that your mitochondria use to make energy—the adenosine triphosphate (ATP) generated by the Krebs Cycle that you probably learned about in high school. *Fat* is the body's second choice for generating cellular energy. *Protein* is the most rarely used fuel since we need its amino acids for building and maintaining structural components of the body like cells, connective tissue, bone, and muscle. Turning protein into glucose to feed into the Krebs Cycle is like feeding your furniture to the woodstove to keep warm. It's only worthwhile in the most dire, life-threatening circumstances when no other macronutrients are available.

Proteins are made from chains of amino acids. They are the building blocks of your cells, and indispensable to life. Were you to go down in a plane crash and find yourself in the Yukon during winter, for instance, you might be able to trap some scrawny rabbits for dinner. *But no matter how many you ate, the paradox is that you would still starve to death*. This is actually called rabbit starvation.

How's that, you ask?

Well, scrawny rabbits lack fat, so the major energy source available from eating them is protein. It turns out that it takes so much metabolic energy to burn protein and convert it to glucose to feed into the Krebs Cycle that the amount of energy available from the lean protein is simply insufficient to sustain life.

This example points to the obvious fact that the nutritional dogma stating that a calorie is just a calorie no matter where it comes from is flat-out wrong.

Calorie charts don't tell you how many calories you have to burn to actually absorb and use the calories in the food. To complicate matters even more, the kind of bacteria you have in your gut also affects how much of a food's potential caloric energy is available to you.

> The reason why low-carb weight-loss diets are heavy on protein, at least in the first phase, is that you can eat a lot of it without utilizing all its calories. *Protein, therefore, is the ultimate skinny food.*

The ultra-low-fat diets espoused by Ornish, Esselstyn, McDougall, and Campbell, for example, limit fat to 10 percent of daily caloric intake. Proteins make up 20 percent to 25 percent of the diet, and carbs take the cake (well, maybe the rice cake) at 65 to 70 percent of caloric intake. The Zone diet recommends 30 percent fat, 30 percent protein, and 40 percent carbs. The New Atkins Diet is the highest in fat of all—as much as 65 to 70 percent. According to standard low-fat dogma, that much fat ought to kill you or at least make you fat. The only hitch is that it doesn't appear to do either one as long as you eat plenty of fiber.

Just a few years ago, like the majority of health professionals, I was still on the low-fat-for-all bandwagon. At the most basic level, I simply assumed that eating fat would make you fat. The logic of that argument is that a gram of protein or carbohydrate has only 4 calories, while a gram of fat has 9. On the other hand, Americans eat much more carbohydrate-rich food than they do fat—low-quality, low-fiber, high-GI (glycemic index) carbs in particular. And since refined carbs cause cravings, eating them leads to eating more overall, which packs on the pounds.

> Think about the low-quality, fat-free foods that get advertised as naturally low fat. Marshmallows, anyone? Gluten-free bakery products? They may not have any gluten, but most of them are still junk food.

Avoiding fat, however, has been so ingrained into public consciousness that eating it can be downright scary for some of us. If you eat too much fat, especially saturated fat, won't your cholesterol go up and give you heart disease? That's what Gordon and I were concerned about when an ultra-low-fat diet didn't work for us, and we experimented with a high-fat, low-carb diet instead. I could literally write a whole book on what I learned about good fats and bad fats, but I'll restrain myself and synthesize some of what I've learned into the next small Science Bite.

CHAPTER 4

The Fat and Cholesterol War

"If you're afraid of butter, use cream."

— JULIA CHILD

Nowhere does nutritional controversy rage more fiercely than in the fat wars. Every time a lipid biochemist—an integrative physician who focuses on prevention, diet, and lifestyle rather than on treating everything with pills—or rogue nutritionist suggests that it might be okay, or even healthy, to eat saturated fats and foods containing cholesterol, they get pounced upon and flattened.

But they keep right on getting up again.

When neurologist David Perlmutter, M.D., wrote about the saturated fat and cholesterol controversy in his best-selling book *Grain Brain*, he did a good job exonerating cholesterol, citing an excellent range of research. His premise was that cholesterol is a necessary nutrient and that the real culprits in cardiovascular disease and Alzheimer's are gluten and carbohydrates.

James Hamblin, M.D., (the health editor of *The Atlantic* magazine) wrote a rebuttal entitled "This Is Your Brain on Gluten."

Hamblin's tagline reads: "The idea that gluten and carbohydrates are at the root of Alzheimer's disease, anxiety, depression, and ADHD has now reached millions of people. It is the basis of a number one bestseller written by a respected physician. What is it worth?"[1]

Hamblin questioned some of the research studies that Perlmutter cited, some of which were indeed—and inevitably—stronger than others. Perlmutter, to his credit, posts many of the studies he cited on his website (www.drperlmutter.com) as free PDFs. I applaud this, since it helps us all increase our nutritional literacy.

The subject of cholesterol is where Hamblin became most vehement. Perlmutter vindicates cholesterol as a villain. In fact, he sings its praises and castigates the use of statins (drugs that prevent the synthesis of cholesterol and thus lower its levels in the body) instead. Ergo, according to the conservative medical establishment, Perlmutter could be killing people with his advice. But the cholesterol story is changing . . . and fast.

Who's right here?

The Redemption of Cholesterol?

Before you begin reading this section, I want to stress two points. First, I'm not a physician and don't give medical advice. Second, I believe that finding your optimal cholesterol intake requires testing and personalization in collaboration with a physician. One size does not fit all.

It's clear that we're in the midst of a sea change concerning ideas about cholesterol, and the entire field is rife with confusion. The way that our bodies process cholesterol differs according to our genetic profile. The expression of our genes, in turn, is affected by what we eat. For example, I can eat all the saturated fat and cholesterol in the world and my LDL-C (concentration of low-density cholesterol, often called "bad cholesterol") remains low. My husband, Gordon, on the other hand, is saturated fat and cholesterol sensitive. His LDL-C rises when he eats foods containing saturated fat and cholesterol.

What we don't know at this point is how cholesterol levels actually relate to heart disease. One school of thought (the old school) is still very concerned with LDL-C. Another school of thought (the new school) views cholesterol as an essential nutrient unrelated to heart disease unless it is oxidized.

What researchers from both schools seem to agree on is that the most important measure of cholesterol in terms of heart disease risk is the total number of small LDL particles (LDL-P). If these particles are oxidized, then they stick to the endothelium (the inside layer of cells) within blood vessels and initiate the process of plaque formation. Since there's no commercially available test for oxidized cholesterol that your doctor can order, at this point, having a high cholesterol particle number (LPL-P) has to be considered a risk factor for coronary artery disease.

The new school of cholesterol points out that cholesterol's critical role in the body has been almost completely ignored, and that it has been cast as a villain on the basis of poor-quality observational studies linking it to heart disease. So first let's take a look at their criticism of the observational cholesterol studies; then we'll review the importance of cholesterol to health.

Chapter 10 will give you the lowdown on observational studies. For now, let's say that a fire is burning down your house. Fortunately, several members of the fire department show up to put out the blaze. An observational study looks at all the things common to fires and comes to the conclusion that firemen cause fires since they're frequently present at the scene—but this is obviously a faulty conclusion. *An observational study can show that firemen are associated with fires, but not that they cause them.*

Cholesterol *is* associated with heart disease (it's found in the fatty plaque inside diseased coronary blood vessels), but that doesn't mean that it *causes* heart disease. Other factors (like oxidation, for example) may be the causal factor. It's just too soon to tell since the story continues to evolve.

What we do know is that cholesterol is absolutely critical to the function of the body. It's a precursor to steroid hormones, including glucocorticoids (anti-inflammatory hormones like cortisol); mineralocorticoids that control salt and water balance; and sex hormones, including androgens, estrogens, and progesterone. Furthermore, cholesterol levels are related to mood.

Twenty-five years ago, when I was still running a mind-body clinic at a Harvard Medical School teaching hospital, there was already research indicating that men with low cholesterol levels were more likely to be depressed than those with higher cholesterol levels. More data of that sort continues to be published.

But much of the mainstream medical community still holds fast to the dogma that saturated fat is bad because it raises cholesterol levels, which in turn increases the risk of cardiovascular disease. The problem with that point of view is that it's been proven wrong again and again. Contrary to what you might think, there's no reliable research that actually supports it. The entire cholesterol hypothesis rests on scanty data indeed, much of it the kind of observational studies that can't establish causation.

A New Look at the Saturated Fat and Cholesterol Dogma

The standard dogma is this: Saturated fat increases cholesterol, which increases cardiovascular disease risk. Ergo, don't eat foods containing saturated fat.

The opponents of this dogma make the point that saturated fat does *not* affect cholesterol levels in 75 percent of people. I'm one of them. The 25 percent that do respond to dietary cholesterol are called hyper-responders. My husband, Gordon, is one of the latter.

But whether or not your body makes cholesterol out of saturated fat, many people don't realize that much of the saturated fat in our bodies doesn't come from eating fat. It comes from eating carbohydrates. Surprised?

> Many people don't realize that much of the saturated fat in our bodies doesn't come from eating fat. It comes from eating carbohydrates.

Dr. Richard Feinman, in the department of cell biology at SUNY Downstate Medical Center, reviewed research advances in saturated fat and health that were presented in May of 2009 at a scientific meeting that addressed the controversy over whether saturated fats are bad or not. According to Feinman:

> A low carbohydrate diet that is high in saturated fat may actually lead to a reduction in plasma saturated fat compared to one that is also high in carbohydrate, a consequence of reduction of triglycerides in the low carbohydrate diet and persistent de novo fatty acid synthesis in the high carbohydrate diet.[2]

Chris Kresser, a practitioner of integrative medicine and much-cited expert (even by Hamblin), cites a meta-analysis of 17 low-carb diet studies involving over 1,100 obese patients published in the journal *Obesity Reviews*. The study found that "low-carb diets were associated with significant decreases in body weight as well as improvement in several CV risk factors, including decrease in triglycerides, fasting glucose, blood pressure, body mass index, abdominal circumference, plasma insulin and c-reactive protein, as well as an increase in HDL cholesterol."[3]

Feinman concluded, "For the past 30 or 40 years, dietary saturated fats have attained a poor reputation especially in relation to cardiovascular health; recommendations to reduce consumption persist even in the face of equivocal or contradictory evidence."

He cites a meta-analysis published in the *American Journal of Clinical Nutrition* that was presented at the meeting he was reporting on, showing "no significant evidence for concluding that dietary saturated fat is associated with an increased risk of cardiovascular disease (CVD)."

Dairy consumption, Feinman reported, is associated with *decreases* in cardiovascular disease risk—even full-fat dairy.

The study that Feinman was referring to was published in the *American Journal of Clinical Nutrition* in 2010. It was a large meta-analysis of prospective studies (the gold standard of how to do a study, as you'll learn about in the Science Bite entitled "How Scientific Is Science?"). Overall the study looked at results involving 347,747 participants, followed for 5 to 23 years. The authors found "no significant evidence for concluding that dietary saturated fat is associated with an increased risk of CHD or CVD. More data are needed to elucidate whether CVD risks are likely to be influenced by the specific nutrients used to *replace* saturated fat."[4] (The italics are mine.)

What nutrients are used to replace saturated fat? Refined carbs, of course. You already know that these spike blood sugar, leading to oxidation, inflammation, glycation, nutrient insufficiency, and gut dysbiosis—the Five Pillars of Dietary Doom.

Shifting the Blame from Fats to Carbs

The bottom line here is that a diet high in *both* fats and carbs is a double whammy. Excess carbohydrates are converted into fat for storage—the de novo fatty acid synthesis that Feinman refers to.

> It's fascinating to realize that a high-carb diet is actually a high-fat diet.

Add more fat to that and, as you'll discover in later chapters, your metabolism will go out of whack. Human beings did not evolve to eat a diet rich in refined carbohydrates. The de novo fatty acid synthesis that follows gives birth to the two-headed monster of obesity and diabetes.

Feinman and other researchers also make the important point that *all saturated fats may not be created equal.* Depending on their chain length, they are likely to have a variety of different biological functions. The problem here is twofold: First, we've oversimplified the story on fats. Second, the story is still unfolding as the field of lipid biochemistry gets increasingly more sophisticated.

You might enjoy watching the video that Peter Attia, M.D., posted on his blog The Eating Academy. It's titled *The Limits of*

Scientific Evidence and the Ethics of Dietary Guidelines—60 Years of Ambiguity (http://vimeo.com/45485034). The video features a masterful analysis of the major studies and governmental decisions that led our country down the low-fat, high-carb path to obesity and chronic illness.

The Eating Academy website also has a comprehensive glossary section. If you look up *triglyceride,* you can read this research summary by Dr. Attia:

> Contrary to what people think, eating saturated fat does not increase saturated fatty acid content in triglycerides. In fact, reduction in carbohydrate intake, coupled with increased saturated fat intake, actually lowers both circulating triglycerides and the amount of saturated fatty acid within triglycerides. Unfortunately, most doctors don't realize this and they tell patients with elevated triglycerides to reduce fat intake. Ironically, this is the wrong treatment.[5]

So what's the bottom line? That's for you and your doc to discover. But one thing is clear. Eating a diet low in carbs (and in Chapter 18 you'll find some of the tests your doc can order to help you figure out how many carbs are right for you) will reduce your circulating saturated fat levels. That may or may not impact your cholesterol, depending on genetic factors. But what's most important is this:

> Try to avoid meals that are high in both saturated fat and refined carbohydrates. It's best to eat that burger—if you eat them—without the bun.

CHAPTER 5

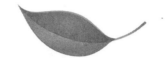

Banish Bad Fats

"You are what what you eat eats."

— MICHAEL POLLAN

Think for a moment about where the fats you eat come from. My friend Lee McCormick owns a grass-fed cattle ranch. His contented cows graze all day long on the succulent Tennessee grasses and are moved frequently to different pastures. The rotation from field to field not only encourages the grasses to grow more lushly but also provides a range of micronutrients to the cows since each pasture has a slightly different plant composition. If you were to eat meat from one of these cows, it would contain healthy fat, rich in omega-3 fatty acids.

Now think of a cow that's raised on a factory farm. When it's time to fatten them up for slaughter, they're moved into pens and fed grain. Since cows evolved to eat grass, they can't digest grain well. That makes them sick. And since they're crowded together, they need antibiotics to reduce the risk of infection. In most cases their feed comes from pesticide-drenched crops including cottonseed—the most highly sprayed crop in the world. Pesticides and pollutants are fat soluble. If you eat meat from one of these animals, its fat is a concentrated source of pesticide residues. It also contains less omega-3 fatty acids and more omega-6 fatty acids (we'll be discussing these in the next chapter).

If you're an omnivore, which meat would you rather eat?

Even if you're a vegan whose fat comes from plants instead of animal products, some fats come from better sources than others. Most oils extracted from seeds—common oils like sunflower-seed oil, canola oil, safflower oil, and the like—are done so under high heat or with chemical solvents. These oxidize the oil, which make it inflammatory. That's why it's wise to choose oils that are both organic *and* cold pressed. The latter process squeezes the oils from the seed without heat so that it doesn't get denatured (oxidized).

In this chapter, we'll take a closer look at fats—from what they are to how to choose the ones best for your health.

What Is a Fat, Anyway?

In order to understand more about good and bad fats, we need to start with a short chemistry lesson. When the doctor tells you that your triglycerides or blood fats are high, what does that actually mean?

A triglyceride looks like the letter *E*. The backbone of the E is a molecule called glycerol. The three bars of the E are made from fatty acids, of which there are many sorts—saturated and unsaturated differing in size and chain length.

The chain of carbon atoms in a fatty acid molecule can vary from as short as 4 to longer than 22. There are four categories: short-chain fatty acids of less than 8 carbons; medium-chain fatty acids of 8 to 14 carbons; long-chain fatty acids of 16 to 20 carbons; and very-long-chain fatty acids of more than 22 carbons. If you're hungry for more information, you'll find a good discussion by Joseph Mercola, D.O., at http://articles.mercola.com/sites/articles/archive/2011/11/11/everything-you-need-to-know-about-fatty-acids.aspx.

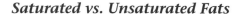

Saturated vs. Unsaturated Fats

If a fatty acid is *saturated*, it means that every carbon atom in the chain is bonded to two hydrogen atoms, protecting it from marauding free radicals on the prowl to steal electrons. If a fatty acid is monounsaturated (*mono* means "one") like the majority of the fat in olive oil, it has one carbon-to-carbon double bond. Two of its carbons are bonded to each other rather than to hydrogen, leaving the fatty acid open to oxidation. If a fatty acid is polyunsaturated (*poly* means "many") it has two or more double bonds and is correspondingly more likely to become oxidized.

The melting point of a fat is determined both by chain length and saturation. Fats like butter, coconut oil, and lard are solid at room temperature because almost all their double bonds are saturated, meaning they're bonded to hydrogen atoms that make the molecules stable. You can leave butter out on the counter for a long time and it won't go rancid, while polyunsaturated fats (or PUFAs) with two or more double bonds are unstable and lose their electrons to free radicals much more easily. Remember this: *When they are oxidized, fats become inflammatory.*

Trans Fats

Without going all wonky on you, suffice it to say that the double bonds of an unsaturated fatty acid can exist in two configurations—cis or trans. Cis is what we most often find in nature; trans is what we find when a PUFA is hydrogenated industrially to saturate the double bonds. The process of hydrogenation turns liquid oils into margarine or the kind of white shortening my mother once used to make piecrusts.

I remember the days when health-conscious folks bought soybean or safflower oil margarine in the belief that it was better than butter. Those mistaken days are gone for good—an example of yesterday's elixir of life turning into today's bad news.

A large body of research demonstrates that artificially produced trans fats are the worst fats of all. They raise bad cholesterol and lower good cholesterol, and although this may or may not have any bearing on heart disease, trans fats do increase the incidence of cardiovascular disease.

Commercial baked goods and processed foods with a long shelf life (basically mummified) owe that dubious distinction to trans fats, which at the time of this writing were on their way to being banned by the Food and Drug Administration (FDA). FDA commissioner Margaret Hamburg stated that reduction of trans fats could prevent "20,000 heart attacks and 7,000 deaths from heart disease each year . . ."[1]

> There are a variety of different trans fats, however, including *vaccenic acid,* which occurs naturally in the milk and meat of ruminant animals. That kind of trans fat doesn't appear to lead to heart disease, insulin resistance, or inflammation and may even have health benefits.[2]

The Polyunsaturated Fat (PUFA) Story

Polyunsaturated fatty acids have a long record of being recommended as heart healthy. That recommendation turns out to be one of the biggest medical research blunders in nutritional history. Let's start with a few facts and figures to put that myth—and the controversy that still surrounds it—into perspective.

The average American of my grandparents' generation (100 years ago) consumed about a pound of vegetable oil annually. Average consumption has now swelled to a whopping 75 pounds per year. We're basically drowning in the stuff. When I first came across this data, it seemed so outlandish I thought it had to be mistaken. But a quick look at the U.S. Department of Agriculture

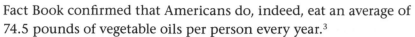

Fact Book confirmed that Americans do, indeed, eat an average of 74.5 pounds of vegetable oils per person every year.[3]

So what's the big deal?, you might ask. Don't PUFAs come from vegetables and lower so-called bad cholesterol? They do, but here's the scoop. Corn, soy, canola, soybean, safflower, sunflower, and grapeseed oils, to name just a few, are all high in PUFAs known as *omega-6 fatty acids.* This class of unsaturated fats comprises fatty acids of different carbon-chain lengths and degrees of unsaturation. What they all have in common is a carbon-to-carbon double bond in what's called the n-6 position of the molecule. Thus the name omega-6 fatty acid.

Omega-6 Fatty Acids

Omega-6 fatty acids are necessary for life. They're deemed *essential fatty acids* because the body can't make them. They have to come from the food we eat. Omega-6 fatty acids are crucial to growth and development, to brain health, and to the health of your hair, bones, skin, and reproductive system. They're also precursors necessary to the synthesis of hormones, a major building block of cell membranes, and a component of LDL particles.

But remember: *Unsaturated fatty acids are inherently unstable and easily oxidized. When the omega-6 fatty acids in LDL particles go rancid (oxidized), the particles become atherogenic. That means that they unleash a cascade of immune reactivity that leads to hardening of the arteries, increasing the risk of heart attack and stroke. People with high levels of oxidized LDL are four times more likely to have a heart attack than those with low-oxidized LDL.*

Although this information has been known by scientists for over 30 years, it's just now getting enough popular press that consumers and their docs are starting to form a new picture of heart health.

Please note that the word on what causes heart disease changes month by month as the old cholesterol dogma slowly goes by the wayside, so stay tuned for the latest news. This can be frustrating because of all the disagreement, so you and your doc need to come to terms over what the best strategy is if you have heart disease.

Oxidized PUFAs

Now that you know a little bit about polyunsaturated fats and oxidation, let's take a quick look at a by-product of the oxidation process. When PUFAs are oxidized, a product known as 4-hydroxy-2-nonenal (4-HNE) is produced. In small quantities 4-HNE has a hormetic effect. *Hormesis* refers to a health-enhancing effect that some poisons have in very small quantities. For example, small amounts of HNEs perform important signaling functions between cells in your body.

In larger concentrations, however, 4-HNE is a toxin. It's a major player in metabolic problems like the development of insulin resistance, neurodegenerative diseases, and cancer because of its propensity to create oxidative stress and inflammation, as well as its involvement in pathways involving both cell proliferation and cell death.[4]

It doesn't take much imagination to realize that increasing intake of vegetable oils rich in omega-6 PUFAs from 1 pound to 75 pounds annually might create a serious toxic overload.

Drowning in Damaged Oil?

But wait a minute here. Perhaps you're wondering, as I did, who on earth could possibly consume 75 pounds a year of PUFAs. That's a whole lot of salad dressing and cooking oil. The answer is that vegetable oils are present in many more products than you might think.

> When you master the art of habitually reading labels, you'll find omega-6 oils in products ranging from baked goods to chips to processed "cheeses," many of which contain no cheese at all. They're chemical concoctions of whey protein and cheap oils. I used to wonder how pizza, covered with real mozzarella cheese, could be sold so cheaply in fast-food chains and supermarkets. The answer is that it can't be.

There *is* no free lunch. Restaurants are in business to make money, so if food prices seem too good to be true, watch out. What's being sold is not likely to be real food at all. Fake food is cheap to produce—although in the long run it's extremely expensive to consume. It can cost you your health, your savings, and eventually your life.

While we're on the subject of bad fats, I have to tell you a little bit more about cottonseed oil. Not only is it rich in omega-6 PUFAs, it's also extracted from the most insecticide-ridden crop on earth. According to the Organic Trade Association:

> Cotton is considered the world's "dirtiest" crop due to its heavy use of insecticides. . . . Cotton covers 2.5 percent of the world's cultivated land yet uses 16 percent of the world's insecticides, more than any other single major crop. . . . Aldicarb, cotton's second best-selling insecticide and most acutely poisonous to humans, can kill a man with just one drop absorbed through the skin, yet it is still used in 25 countries and the US, where 16 states have reported it in their groundwater.[5]

Cottonseed meal, hulls, and whole seeds are also commonly used as animal feed. The insecticide residues are stored in the fat of the animals and show up in their meat and milk. When we consume these animal-derived foods, the insecticides are passed on to us and stored in our fat. If you nurse a baby, it travels from your fat to theirs.

Still think that it's too expensive to give your children organic milk—that is, if you give them milk at all? Please, moms. If your kids eat dairy, make sure that it's from pasture-raised cows and guaranteed organic. And if your kids eat cheese, make sure that it's real cheese made from the milk of pasture-raised cows, goats, or sheep and not an imitation cheese food made from vegetable oil.

In Part III, you'll start your PlantPlus lifestyle conversion by cleansing your kitchen and tossing all the polyunsaturated vegetable oils in the trash. If you're used to using these in baking, substitute cold-pressed organic coconut oil, cold-pressed organic avocado oil, or butter instead. If you use them for sautéing, substitute cold-pressed, organic extra-virgin olive oil. Beware, since many cheap supermarket omega-6 oils (often extracted with organic solvents like hexane and loaded with insecticide residues) are labeled so that you can easily mistake them for olive oil unless you read the label with care.

Eliminating bad fats and using good fats is key to a PlantPlus lifestyle. In the next chapter, you'll learn more about good fats—what they are and why they're healthy.

CHAPTER 6

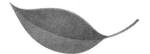

Cherish Good Fats

"You, as a food buyer, have the distinct privilege of proactively participating in shaping the world your children will inherit."

— JOEL SALATIN, *HOLY COWS AND HOG HEAVEN:*
THE FOOD BUYER'S GUIDE TO FARM FRIENDLY FOOD

Chickens raised outside in a pasture get to scratch around in the dirt, eat insects, gobble up worms, and hobnob happily with their flock. The eggs laid by these back-to-the-earth mama hens have a better fat composition than factory-farmed eggs, including as much as 20 times more healthful omega-3 fatty acids.

But when you buy a dozen eggs at the store—eggs marked "natural," "organic," "cage-free," "humanely raised," or "vegetarian"—what does the label promise actually mean? Can you trust those bucolic pictures of hens pecking around the base of a tree, or does "cage-free" mean theoretical access to the outside through a tiny door that's rarely used? Does vegetarian feed consist of pesticide-ridden cottonseed hulls or meal? The word *natural* is meaningless, as there are no regulations that back it up. The word *organic*, on the other hand, is tightly regulated.

But we also need to consider ethical realities. A hen who eats organic food but lives as a debeaked prisoner in a crowded cage is not a happy camper.

A website called Cornucopia has an egg-rating system that considers nutritional and ethical questions (www.cornucopia.org /organic-egg-scorecard). A 5-egg rating is "exemplary," generally given to eggs from small- to medium-scale family farms where hens enclosed in mobile pens are rotated frequently to fresh pasture. A 1-egg rating, in contrast, generally refers to store-brand or private-label eggs rated as "ethically deficient." Cornucopia explains, "Our research indicates that the vast majority of organic eggs for private label brands are produced on industrial farms that house hundreds of thousands of birds and do not grant the birds meaningful outdoor access."

I believe that it's our responsibility to treat animals kindly, a civil rights issue that's inspiring more conscious food choices by younger consumers and baby boomers alike. We vote for the state of animals and for our own health through what we buy.

Although a dozen eggs from our local family farm costs about $7.99—more than double the price of other "premium" organic-looking eggs—we bite the bullet and buy the ethical eggs. It was a shock to read on the Cornucopia site that Whole Foods 365 Organic brand eggs get only a 1-egg rating. They're factory farmed, as are eggs from Trader Joe's, the Safeway Organics line, Eggland's Best, and dozens of other brands—some of which are even labeled as if they come from family farms.

If you do choose to eat ethical eggs, one thing you can be sure of is that they contain a wealth of good fats for you. As food guru Michael Pollan says, "You are what what you eat eats." So let's turn our attention to which fats are good for us to eat and why that's so.

Omega-3 Fatty Acids

We hear all the time that we ought to eat fatty fish—that two servings a week will actually prolong life. The health benefits, as you'll find out momentarily, really are impressive. My mother loved canned salmon and sardines so much that one or the other was almost always her go-to food at lunchtime. If you're fortunate enough to like canned sardines, they're a very convenient source of omega-3s. They're also an environmentally sustainable choice. Sardines are small fish; there's an abundant supply in the wild; and because they're near the bottom of the food chain, their mercury content is low.

> Omega-3 fatty acids are essential for life and have to come from diet since the body has a very limited ability to manufacture them. *These fatty acids are potent anti-inflammatories in blood vessels, joints, and elsewhere throughout the body.* They can lower triglycerides and blood pressure. You may also have read about their use to alleviate depression, treat rheumatoid arthritis, and help with a variety of other conditions.

Just as omega-6 fatty acids are named for where in the carbon chain unsaturated double bonds occur, so are omega-3 fatty acids. I'll spare you the details. There are, however, several types of omega-3 fatty acids that vary in chain length and degree of unsaturation. Two types of omega-3s—EPA (eicosapentaenoic acid) and DHA (docosahexaenoic acid)—occur primarily in fish, but there are vegetable sources as well. Vegans can get DHA from marine algae supplements. EPA can be made by the body in very small quantities from ALA (alpha-linolenic acid) found in walnuts, flax, chia, and hemp seeds.

While there's no controversy about whether omega-3s are good for you, there is a controversy about how much omega-6 versus omega-3 fatty acids you need to keep your body healthy. The majority of people, as you now know, consume about 75 times more vegetable oil rich in omega-6 fatty acids than their grandparents or great-grandparents did. At the same time, the great majority of

Americans consume too little healthful omega-3 fatty acids either from fatty fish, algae supplements, or krill or fish oil supplements.

The result is that the balance of our fatty acids, at least according to some experts, is seriously off kilter. Most integrative medical professionals will tell you that the ratio of omega-6 to omega-3 fatty acids should be 1:1, or at most 4:1. In contrast, the typical American diet has a ratio that approximates 20:1.

Conventional nutrition researchers and government agencies vociferously disagree, possibly because the *PUFAS-are-healthy-so-eat-a-lot-of-them myth* persists in the face of excellent data to the contrary.

The AHA Eats Their Words

The American Heart Association has had to eat their recommendations repeatedly on what kind of dietary fat we should be eating. The latest episode (which is being hotly debated by both sides) was in 2013, when an article published in *BMJ*, the *British Medical Journal,* demonstrated that instructing men with heart disease to replace saturated fat with polyunsaturated fatty acids (PUFAs) rich in omega-6 fatty acids increased their rate of death from all causes, including cardiovascular disease.[1]

An article about the *BMJ* study appeared in *Science Daily*, a website that covers the latest research news. The reporter noted this:

The most common dietary PUFA in Western diets is omega-6 linoleic acid (n-6 LA for short). UK dietary recommendations are cautious about high intakes of omega-6 PUFAs, but some other health authorities, including the American Heart Association, have recently repeated advice to maintain, and even to increase, intake of omega-6 PUFAs. This has caused some controversy, because evidence that linoleic acid lowers the risk of cardiovascular disease is limited.[2]

The article goes on to quote one of the authors of the *BMJ* study who argues against the "saturated fat bad, omega-6 PUFA good" dogma and suggests politely that the American Heart Association guidelines on omega-6 PUFAs may be misguided. The authors also "underscore the need to properly align dietary advice and recommendations with the scientific evidence base."

> As many experts who have carefully evaluated the data on saturated fats agree, the American Heart Association's insistence that saturated fats are bad and PUFAs are good is based on a scanty and suspect scientific database. Nonetheless, it's a health dogma that has been excruciatingly slow to die.

When the *BMJ* article was published, the blogosphere resounded with salvos from both sides of the polyunsaturated-fat fence. "The article is suspect." "No, it's the Holy Grail—one more nail in the PUFA coffin." What's the bottom line? Research studies need to be replicated to make sure that associations haven't appeared by chance, and to rule out a variety of other errors. That takes time. So for now the fat wars continue to rage.

Just as I was putting the finishing touches on this book, a small crack in the low-fat wall finally opened. The 2013 guidelines on cholesterol, blood pressure, and obesity management compiled by the National Heart, Lung, and Blood Institute (NHLBI) reversed the recommendation to lower fat intake overall. The NHLBI lifestyle recommendations are now more in line with a Mediterranean-type diet based on plants, some whole grains, and healthy fats, including olive oil, nuts, seeds, fish oil, and avocados.

Let's take a closer look at some of the good fats.

Olive Oil

I consider olive oil a Superfood. It's a monounsaturated fatty acid (MUFA), so it's more stable and less prone to oxidation than the PUFAs. A Mediterranean diet, arguably one of the healthiest diets overall, is rich both in olive oil and in omega-3s from seafood. Olive oil is not only healthful, as we'll review in a minute, but also intoxicatingly fragrant and delicious. It adds a subtle, sweet-earthy flavor to whatever foods you add it to.

But it's important to distinguish between real and fake, good and bad, olive oils.

You need to read the fine print on the label to see what you've got. Fake olive oils abound in supermarkets. They're bottled and labeled to appear like olive oil but may be a blend of olive oil and PUFAs, or the olive oil may have been industrially produced using poisonous solvents to leach out the oil, which denatures it. The rancid oil is then deodorized. The resultant "olive oil" has no redeeming features. Instead it promotes inflammation.

Look for *organic, cold-pressed extra-virgin olive oil.* Instead of being extracted with chemical solvents, this kind of oil is mechanically pressed from the olives in a process that doesn't oxidize the oil. The unfiltered variety of cold-pressed oil is cloudy and contains a little sediment. The filtered variety is clear. Either one is great. I suggest buying the best olive oil that your budget can handle, and buying it in glass bottles rather than plastic, since chemicals from the plastic can leach into the oil.

People who consume olive oil as a steady feature of their diet are less likely to develop cardiovascular disease, including stroke, high blood pressure, high cholesterol levels, and high triglycerides. Olive oil also helps preserve the endothelial layer (the inside lining) of blood vessels and reduce inflammation, which may be part of the way it prevents the buildup of plaque and fights hardening of the arteries.

Olive oil is also high in a substance called hydroxytyrosol, which is being explored at Houston Methodist Hospital as a preventative for breast cancer in a high-risk group of women. An article in *Medical News Today* sums up some important research on olive oil on the possible prevention and treatment of breast cancer:

> The researchers decoded a complete cascade of signals within the cells of breast tumors that are activated by virgin olive oil. They concluded that the oil reduces the activity of p21Ras, an oncogene, prevents DNA damage, encourages tumor cell death, and triggers changes in protein signaling pathways. The team found that while corn oil—which is rich in n-6 polyunsaturated fatty acids—increased the aggressiveness of tumors, virgin olive oil had the opposite effect.[3]

The MUFAs in extra-virgin olive oil (EVOO) also help regularize carbohydrate metabolism and dampen down spikes in blood sugar, which, as you know, will help reduce the nasty trio of dietary demons—glycation, inflammation, and oxidation. That said, I'll end this accolade to the olive with a reminder that although olive oil is practically a magic potion, it's not a substitute for medical care.

Coconut Oil

I turned on CNN one day and there was Chief Medical Correspondent Sanjay Gupta, M.D., looking squirrelly. He was reporting on the purported health benefits of coconut oil despite the fact that it is a—perish the thought for conventional medicine—saturated fat. He concluded that it didn't seem to be as bad as some other saturated fats.

The fact is that despite extravagant claims for the health benefits of coconut oil—from lessening symptoms of Alzheimer's disease to promoting weight loss—there are very few studies that have been done to support the largely anecdotal health claims made about this "miracle oil."

Coconut oil is more saturated, and thus more stable against oxidation, compared to other oils. While coconut oil is 92 percent saturated, butter is only 63 percent saturated, while olive oil trails at 15 percent saturation. The kind of saturated fat in coconut oil is also unusual. It's a medium-chain fatty acid (MCT) rather than a long-chain fatty acid. Because MCTs are transported directly to the liver, they are burned as fuel very quickly and may raise metabolic rate slightly. In other words, this is a fat that might help make you skinny. At least that's the word on the street. But only one small study of 40 women has been done, and more are needed to validate the weight-loss claims.

Since I've arrived at the point where saturated fat and I have become friends (at least in limited quantities), I use coconut oil in much of my baking. It results in a crispy, tender cookie. And since it's extremely stable with a shelf life of about five years due to its high percentage of saturation, it's less likely to become rancid than other fats. That fact alone makes it a good fat in my book.

Avocados and Avocado Oil

Avocado oil is pressed from the fruit of the avocado, not the seed. Avocado flesh, as well as its oil, has abundant phytochemicals and vitamins, including A, B_1, B_2, pantothenic acid, vitamins E and D, and other micronutrients. It also contains several plant sterols that reduce inflammation. Research has also demonstrated that avocados contain several powerful antioxidants that limit the activity of free radicals.

Avocados are also *extremely* rich in fiber—about 10 grams to one fruit.

So, harkening back to the Five Pillars of Dietary Doom, avocados are a big winner. They:

1. Reduce inflammation

2. Reduce oxidative stress

3. Provide micronutrients

4. Nourish gut microbes with their fiber

5. Help normalize blood sugar and reduce glycation by slowing the absorption of carbohydrates

We eat avocados several times a week, adding them to salads often. Gordon also makes spectacular guacamole—a marvelous snack to scoop up with celery, carrots, jicama, or lettuce leaves.

Extra-virgin avocado oil, like olive oil, is high in monounsaturated fats, has a high smoke point so that you can use it to sauté foods, and tastes great. Depending on the brand, some avocado oils are also a good source of the vitamin CoQ_{10}, or ubiquinol, so important for heart health.

$\emptyset \emptyset \emptyset$

So now you've got the word on bad and good fats. To sum it all up:

- Fats are only as good as the plants or animals they come from. Choose cold-pressed extra-virgin olive, avocado, or coconut oil; and eat eggs, dairy, and meat that come from humanely raised, pasture-fed animals. Eat wild-caught fish that are low in mercury because they're small or Alaskan wild-caught salmon.

- According to the latest research, saturated fats are good for most people, while the supposedly heart-healthy PUFAs are not. Beware, since your doctor (or your body) may not agree.

Now that we've safely traversed the turbulent World of Fat, it's time to turn our attention to the equally contentious and controversial World of Grain. Once you know what the grain flap is all about, then you'll be in a better position to determine whether or not grains are a Plus food for your personalized nutritional profile.

CHAPTER 7

Grain Brain, Wheat Belly, and Paleo Pigs

"Nobody is qualified to become a statesman who is entirely ignorant of the problem of wheat."

— SOCRATES

A 2005 study out of the Netherlands was conducted to investigate the global pattern of "diseases of affluence," the same chronic health conditions we've been talking about—from diabetes to dementia. The researchers hypothesized that cereal-based diets could be the problem. They studied pigs, not people, but their results were interesting. They fed half the pigs a grain-free diet of the sort that early hunter-gatherer societies would have eaten. In other words, foods that you could hunt, fish, or forage. They fed the other half a "cereal-based swine feed."

The grain-free pigs (I think of them as Paleo Piggies) were the metabolic winners. They had significantly higher insulin sensitivity, lower diastolic blood pressure, and lower levels of C-reactive protein—a powerful measure of inflammation and predictor of heart disease risk. The lower your CRP level, the healthier it is, whether you're a piggy or a person.

Part of the explanation for the adverse effects of the cereal-based swine feed may be due to a class of proteins called *lectins*. While the lectin *gliadin* is found only in wheat, rye, spelt, barley, kamut, and sometimes oatmeal, similar compounds are found in all grains and beans (legumes).

What the Devil Are Lectins?

Lectins are mild toxins, antinutrients that compose part of the innate pest-control system of plants. Unfortunately, we are among the pests that lectins are meant to discourage.

Lectins are proteins that bind to the carbohydrates (sugars) attached to the outer surfaces of the cell membrane. These carbohydrate-binding proteins are very specific. Each one attaches to a distinct sugar, which is a way of recognizing and amplifying a specific chemical signal.

When I worked as a cancer-cell biologist, I used a lectin that is a phytohemagglutinin (a plant molecule that causes red blood cells to clump up) called Concanavalin A (Con A) as a label for certain receptors in the cell membrane. Con A is extracted from jack beans, which are poisonous to humans even when cooked. I remember my postdoctoral professor cautioning me about exposure to the jack bean meal that I was extracting Con A from. The beans can be a deadly poison. So can castor beans, which contain a lectin called *ricin*, one of the deadliest poisons known to man—the stuff of James Bond films and real-life international spy thriller scenarios.

Common edible beans of all types contain lectins with antinutrient properties, many of which are at least mildly toxic. In general, that's not a problem. The response to mildly poisonous elements in our diet is an example of *hormesis*. As I've mentioned, hormesis is a generally favorable biological response to a substance, which, in higher doses, can be poisonous.

Most beans are hormetic rather than overtly poisonous; otherwise, the world's bean-eating populations would be long dead. But every once in a while, a crop of beans has more lectins than usual. A 1999 editorial published in the *British Medical Journal* by allergist David L.J. Freed, "Do Dietary Lectins Cause Disease?," begins with an interesting human anecdote:

> In 1988 a hospital launched a "healthy eating day" in its staff canteen at lunchtime. One dish contained red kidney beans, and 31 portions were served. At 3 pm one of the customers, a surgical registrar, vomited in theatre. Over the next four hours 10 more customers suffered profuse vomiting, some with diarrhoea. All had recovered by next day. No pathogens were isolated from the food, but the beans contained an abnormally high concentration of the lectin phytohaemagglutinin. . . . In the past two decades we have realised that many lectins are (*a*) toxic, inflammatory, or both; (*b*) resistant to cooking and digestive enzymes; and (*c*) present in much of our food.[1]

The highest levels of lectins are found in grains, legumes, dairy, eggs, and the nightshade family (tomatoes, potatoes, green pepper, and eggplant), as well as oils extracted from beans and grains.

Since we are each physiologically unique, we respond to lectins in different ways. People with chronic intestinal inflammation, for example, are particularly sensitive to lectins because the cells of the gut lining are constantly renewing themselves, and the sugar molecules on the surface of immature cells are more likely to bind lectins. Since every cell in the body has sugars that lectins can bind to, they are at least suspects in physiological disruption, although a bean or grain must remain innocent until definitively proven guilty.

David Freed's editorial in the *British Medical Journal* is an old one, published in 1999. It was meant as a heads-up to physicians and introduced many of them to what Freed called "the stone age diet." Freed explained, "The mucus stripping effect of lectins also offers an explanation for the anecdotal finding of many allergists that a 'stone age diet,' which eliminates most starchy foods and therefore most lectins, protects against common upper respiratory viral infections: without lectins in the throat the nasopharyngeal mucus lining would be more effective as a barrier to viruses."

So should we give up all grains, beans, dairy, eggs, chocolate, and most especially ratatouille, a delicious nightshade stew made of tomatoes, green peppers, eggplant, and onions? The Paleo community says we should give up most of those things, as does the macrobiotic community. But what does the scientific data tell us?

Gluten: Wheat Belly and Beyond

Cardiologist William Davis, M.D., author of the best-selling book *Wheat Belly*, makes a compelling case against the protein *gliadin*—a component of gluten—found in wheat and other grains including spelt, rye, barley, kamut, and possibly oatmeal (although to a much smaller degree). Apparently the old strains of wheat had far less gliadin, but newer strains have been carefully selected for better yield, more resistance to drought and pests, and more gluten (yes, that's the stuff that makes a good artisanal bagel so irresistibly chewy). Sigh.

Apparently the wheat of the Bible, the Staff of Life, doesn't bear much resemblance to the overbred and genetically modified wheat that modern agribusiness has bred. Wheat is a seed, and as such it's equipped with its own survival toolkit. It can't get up and run if a hungry predator tries to eat it for lunch. Instead, it has developed toxic lectins, *antinutrients*, to discourage nibblers from eating the grain and thereby reducing the grasses to extinction.

If eating a wild food makes predators sick, they lose their taste for the offending item very quickly. That's the magic of feedback, particularly in the area of food. The problem is that most humans don't know when gliadin or other lectins are making them ill. It's so ubiquitous, and we are so used to feeling however we generally feel, that we don't necessarily associate fatigue, a sore tummy, bloating and gas, headache, muscle pain, or other symptoms with eating gluten.

For example, when my husband, Gordon, and I were on a low-fat diet, we ate a tremendous amount of grain. Yes, it was organic, but oatmeal, whole-wheat pasta, and sprouted whole-grain bread were the staples of our diet.

I felt fatigued and bloated most of the time—as did Gordon—often with stomach cramps. The problem, we were both surprised to discover, was the large amount of grain we'd been consuming. Truth be told, I had a serious bias against all the antigluten articles I'd seen in magazines. It seemed like the new villain du jour, the one-size-fits-all cause of every possible ailment. It seemed that gluten, like soy, had fallen hostage to a few poorly informed, militant writers who grossly exaggerated and bent the facts.

One of my initial thoughts about gluten was, *How bad can it be? After all, only 1 percent of the population actually has a serious autoimmune response to it.* If you are one of them, then you have celiac disease (CD).

Celiac Disease

When I was a child of five or six, I was diagnosed with CD because I complained of bloating and diarrhea. The doctor must have used his imagination to come up with that diagnosis, since an accurate diagnosis of CD back then would have required a biopsy of my small intestine. And I would surely have remembered that!

If you have bona fide CD, the villi of your small intestine (villi are small protuberances that increase the surface area of your intestine so that more nutrients can be absorbed) are partially destroyed by an autoimmune response. Inflammation rules, and you may also be malnourished because the epithelial cells lining the small intestine can't readily absorb nutrients. On the other hand, like 50 percent of people diagnosed with CD, you might not have any gastrointestinal symptoms at all. That's what makes it so hard to diagnose.

I have no recollection of whether or not I'd lost weight as a child, or what other symptoms I might have had, but I was promptly put on a gluten-free diet. As close as memory serves, that involved eating a lot of steak, baked potatoes, and bananas. After several years the whole episode seemed forgotten and I was put back on the Standard American Diet. Apparently I didn't have CD after all, or if I do I still don't know it.

But you may be among the 1 percent of Americans who do have CD. According to the University of Chicago Celiac Disease Center, 3 million Americans are affected. To put that in context, 2.7 million Americans have epilepsy; 30,000 have cystic fibrosis; 1 million have Parkinson's disease; 2.1 million have rheumatoid arthritis; 400,000 have multiple sclerosis.

Since the symptoms of CD are diffuse—ranging from diarrhea to fatigue; fibromyalgia; cognitive deficits, including confusion and "foggy" brain; stomach pains; skin problems; and joint pain—it takes on average four years to be diagnosed. During that time, the disease can cause progressively greater damage and lead to other autoimmune disorders, infertility, osteoporosis, neurological disorders, and even cancer.

When people with celiac disease are put on a gluten-free diet, that means eliminating virtually all foods made from glutenous grains—including malt when it comes from barley (bye-bye, beer)—regardless of whether these foods actually contain gluten.

Every trace of gliadin must be removed from the diet to avoid the autoimmune reaction it causes. It's not enough to put away the bread, beer, and baked goods alone. You'd be surprised by how many foods contain gliadin. Almost every processed food is suspect. Hello, a jar of mustard? A can of soup? Soy sauce? Instant coffee? Communion wafers? You get the drift. It's hidden in almost all processed foods.

The label "gluten-free" has become shorthand for foods that people with CD can safely eat. Most people, however, don't have a serious autoimmune response to gliadin. Nonetheless, they may have an intolerance to gliadin or other proteins in gluten.

Gluten Intolerance

The spectrum of gluten intolerance is just now being investigated. Physicians are clambering for objective scientific criteria to diagnose it, especially since so many patients put themselves on gluten-free diets for no reason other than their bias against it.

A friend of mine hosted a dinner party—not easy in this day and age since people's diets vary so widely. When she asked one of the gluten-free guests why she didn't eat gluten, the guest had no idea whatsoever. She didn't know what gluten was, why it might be bad for her, or what the symptoms of gluten intolerance look like.

An excellent HuffPo article, "50 Shades of Gluten (Intolerance)," by Chris Kresser, a notable Paleo blogger and author of *Your Personal Paleo Code*, sheds some light on gluten intolerance that is not celiac disease. Kresser includes some interesting information on antibodies to proteins in gluten (other than gliadin) that can cause a reaction in people who don't have CD (www.huffingtonpost.com /chris-kresser/gluten-intolerance_b_2964812.htm). Kresser writes:

> CD is just one possible expression of gluten intolerance; there are many other ways that sensitivity to gluten can manifest in the body. These are collectively referred to as "Non-Celiac Gluten Sensitivity," or NCGS. There's no consensus definition of NCGS yet, but the most common understanding is that it's a reaction to gluten that is not autoimmune (like CD) or allergic

(like wheat allergy). Another definition I've seen is, "a reaction to gluten that resolves when gluten is removed from the diet and CD and allergy have been ruled out."[2]

The claim is that as many as 1 in 20 Americans have NCGS, although many conventional physicians don't believe that it exists.

Another interesting overview of gluten intolerance comes from functional medicine physician Mark Hyman, M.D. Its title? *Gluten: What You Don't Know Might Kill You.* In spite of the alarmist tone, it's a good quick review of the field, including some interesting scientific studies (www.youtube.com /watch?v=yLJSmJ0bMlk).

Hyman, Kresser, and essentially all health-care professionals concerned about gluten intolerance recommend taking it out of the diet for two to four weeks and observing what effect its elimination has on your health. Remember, the PlantPlus Diet involves some sleuthing on your part, including the first four weeks— the Reboot—when all grains (and thus all sources of gluten) are eliminated.

When Gordon's cardiologist heard that we were experimenting with our diet by eliminating grains, she immediately thought we were "going Paleo." The Paleolithic diet is very popular with a growing number of adherents, though it's widely suspect in medical circles. Read on and you'll get the drift of this powerful nutritional controversy.

The Paleolithic (Paleo) Diet

Loren Cordain, Ph.D., is an expert in nutrition and exercise physiology. A professor at Colorado State University, his website describes him as the world's foremost authority on "the evolutionary basis of diet and disease." Author of over 100 peer-reviewed journal articles and abstracts, Dr. Cordain's work reached millions of people when his popular book, *The Paleo Diet*, became a blockbuster. You can watch a fascinating academic lecture that Cordain gives on the origin and evolution of the Western diet complete with PowerPoints at www.youtube.com/watch?v=5dw1MuD9EP4.

I'll summarize a few of his main points for you.

Cordain and his colleagues examined ethnographic observations (qualitative cultural reports) of what 229 hunter-gatherer societies ate. There were only 13 quantitative studies documenting the proportions of plants and meat that made up various indigenous diets. Inuit Eskimos from Greenland, for example, ate 96 percent animal food since the growing season is too short to produce much in the way of vegetables. The Nunamiut, an Eskimo group living in northwest Alaska, ate 99 percent animal food. Eliminating these two groups as extreme cases, the other 11 indigenous societies studied averaged two-thirds of their energy intake from meat and the rest from plants.

There were no vegan societies, since, as Cordain succinctly puts it, a vegan diet is lethal unless it's supplemented with vitamin B_{12}. And there were no supplements in Paleolithic times.

Today, grains, dairy, vegetable oil, and sugar compose 79 percent of our energy sources from food.

Our current love affair with grain, according to Cordain, had its roots back in Neolithic times when agricultural societies replaced hunter-gatherer lifestyles. That happened between 5,500 to 10,000 years ago. Since a generation is measured as 33 years, 10,000 years constitutes just 303 generations, not a long time in terms of evolution. Cordain's thesis is that the human genome is relatively stable, so we are not now—nor were we then—genetically suited to be grain eaters.

The Paleo diet is built on a food pyramid that makes most physicians faint with anxiety. The base of the pyramid is pasture-raised lean meat. Wild animals that hunter-gatherers ate would have been extremely lean compared to the corn-fed, fat-marbled meat that most Americans eat. A friend of mine from Israel simply can't abide our factory-farmed meat. She finds it nauseatingly greasy, toxic tasting, and profoundly unappetizing. While my husband, Gordon, and I do eat grass-fed meat (at least when we're home), it's not the bottom of our food pyramid. Vegetables are. But contrary to what many people think, the Paleo diet also involves eating a lot of vegetables.

On the Paleo diet, fruits and vegetables are supposed to costitute 35 percent to 45 percent of daily calories, which adds up to a lot of plants. Next on the Paleo pyramid comes nuts and seeds. Healthy oils like olive oil, coconut oil, and avocados are at the apex.

Does this mean that I support the Paleo diet? As you know, I don't believe that there is any one-size-fits-all diet. While Gordon and I don't eat much grain, we're not "Paleo" eaters. We're "Personalized eaters." When lab tests revealed that both of us had high LDL-P (cholesterol particle numbers), we responded by cutting back on meat. I had noticed that high LDL-P was mentioned by several bloggers on Paleo sites, who had started to wonder whether the diet was causing the problem. The only way to know, of course, is to experiment. That's what diet personalization is all about.

Here's an impromptu gluten experiment that Gordon and I conducted. Small quantities of gluten don't seem to have any immediate effect on either one of us. We can eat a piece of pizza or a crusty roll once in a while when we're out. But one night after almost two years on a 99 percent grain-free diet, we splurged and decided to split a pizza. I was up all night with a painful charley horse in one leg and intense cramping in the other foot. Did the gluten cause these bizarre symptoms? I can't be sure unless the experiment is repeated several times with the same results. But one pain-riddled sleepless night was quite enough for me. I won't be eating that much gluten at one time again.

It's up to every person to experiment with foods mindfully and observe the effects on their immediate state of well-being and also on their lab tests over time.

So what's the gluten bottom line? No matter what our ancestors ate 10,000 years ago, our lives and locales have changed drastically. While our genetic code changes very slowly over millions of years, we can adapt successfully to a variety of new environments because of our *epigenome*, the control panel through which environmental conditions—everything from the food we eat to the stress we experience—change the expression of our genes.

So, no matter what our ancestors ate, it's possible that we can still be healthy eating a different kind of diet. Even dogs, carnivores that they are, adapted to eating starch that they snitched from the camps of our Neolithic, grain-farming ancestors.[3] Some people thrive on a diet containing whole grains. Others don't. On the other hand, refined grain products that send your blood sugar soaring aren't meant to be a major component of either the canine diet or the human diet.

We've opted to feed our two best friends, standard poodles Milo and Mitzi (M and M), a grain-free diet. Too many American companion animals suffer from the same junk food–related diseases as their humans do. They're fat, arthritic, diabetic, and prone to cancer. And where pets are concerned, they're like children. The responsibility for their nutrition lies with the adult humans who care for them. You can feed them the equivalent of American fast food, or you can feed them foods made from animal protein unadulterated with additives like food coloring and preservatives.

When you begin to design your own carb-reasonable Plant-Plus lifestyle, you'll begin with *four weeks* of eliminating all grains. By observing the results, both in your health and well-being and in the medical tests that we'll go over together at the end of Part I, you'll have a good idea of how grains affect you. Because these dietary changes will eliminate blood sugar spikes as well as change the hormones that regulate hunger and satiety, your previous carb cravings will diminish or even disappear. Stay tuned for the reason why in the next Science Bite.

CHAPTER 8

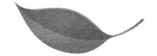

Sugar, Insulin, and Hunger

"How can a nation be called great if its bread tastes like Kleenex?"

— JULIA CHILD

Perhaps we might ask, How can a nation be called great if the people are obese, but still hungry? Why can't we be satisfied anymore? We're like Hungry Ghosts—denizens of a mythical Buddhist realm. These unfortunate beings have tiny mouths and huge bellies, condemning them to a state of perpetual want. Always seeking satisfaction, Hungry Ghosts miss out on being present to the here and now.

Why is that happening? Part of the problem is that we're constantly surrounded by high-carb, high-sugar foods.

> We're constantly surrounded by high-carb, high-sugar foods. You'll find them not only in the supermarket but also in places like the hardware store, the pet-supply store, the toy store, the nail salon, and even vending machines in schools. The simple abundance of crap carbs makes them almost impossible to avoid and very hard to resist.

That brings us to the threefold topic of sugar, insulin (the fat-storing hormone), and leptin (the satiety hormone). It's bad enough to have to watch your weight without much success. But it's brutal to go hungry while that's happening. The PlantPlus Diet is meant to eliminate the double whammy of being fat while going hungry. In order for you to understand how the double whammy works and how to disable it, we'll start by exploring the secret life of sugar.

Glucose

Glucose is a molecule that's both our best friend and our worst enemy. Our bodies run on the stuff. The clever little mitochondria that threw their lot in with ours a couple of million years ago convert glucose to the adenosine triphosphate (ATP) that powers every cell in our body. The clever little mitochondria can also make ATP out of fat.

We're all built like hybrid vehicles that can switch fuel sources when necessary. In times of feasting, we burn glucose. In times of fasting, we burn fat. Insulin is the equivalent of your engine's fuel-selector switch. When insulin levels are high, you burn dietary carbs and store any leftovers as glycogen (a polymer of glucose), or as fat. When insulin levels are low, you burn fat as the fuel of choice.

Metabolic Flexibility

> The ability to burn either carbs or fat for energy, and switch easily between the two, is called *metabolic flexibility*. Making sure that there's energy available not only in times of feast, but also in times of famine, is what metabolic flexibility is all about.

Human beings worldwide have always had to cope with periods of famine brought about by drought, war, winter, or natural disaster. But even in a country as affluent as the United States, poverty still results in what social-service agencies call *food insecurity*. Fifty million Americans, including nearly 17 million children, endure periods when sufficient food may not be available. That's one in six of us. Can you imagine? We have to do better than that.

But for those of us privileged enough to have a steady supply of food, periods of feast and famine most often have a diurnal rhythm. During the day when we're eating, we typically burn off glucose first. During the night when we're fasting, we switch over to fat burning. That's why it's best not to eat after dinner. It's not just the calories that you need to worry about. But don't kid yourself—calories still matter, and grazing your way to the bedroom racks up more of them. How much fat you burn depends in part on the *length* of the evening fast . . . the time until you break fast, or breakfast. The longer the time of fasting between meals, the less insulin you'll secrete and the more fat you'll burn.

The Secret Life of Insulin

Insulin's job is to get glucose out of the blood *pronto*. You can think of glucose—your body's main fuel source—as akin to gasoline. It's great when it's burned for fuel or stored in a container (glycogen or fat) for later use, but it's poisonous when it gets loose and runs amok creating advanced glycation end products. As you already know, AGEs deform proteins, stiffen your tissues, build up as permanent sludge, and create inflammation. They're not what Mother Nature had in mind for you. The body evolved to keep very tight control over blood glucose levels in an environment where refined carbs were rare.

Unfortunately, processed foods made from refined carbs release more sugar than the average person's metabolism can cope with. And I'm not just talking about eating candy and cookies, french fries, ice cream, pasta, and white bread either. *Two slices of whole-wheat bread break down rapidly into two entire tablespoons full of sugar.* That's a big herd of glucose molecules for your insulin to round up and drive inside your cells where they belong.

Both liver and muscle cells convert extra glucose into a starchy chain, or polymer, called *glycogen*. When the body needs more energy, for instance during exercise, glucose is released from glycogen by a hormone called *glucagon*. When a person "hits the wall" at about mile 20 of a marathon, it's because they've used up all their glycogen stores and have to switch over to fat burning.

Since room for glycogen storage is relatively limited, most of the additional fuel you take on at the pump (your daily carb supply) gets stored as fat. Your adipose, or fat tissue, is composed of cells that shrink and swell dependent upon how much triglyceride (the storage form of fat) you have on board at any given time. The liver synthesizes triglycerides, loads them into trucks made of protein, and sends the resulting very low density lipoproteins (VLDLs) out into the blood for immediate delivery to your favorite fat pads.

But glucose isn't the body's only immediate fuel source. We also burn the sugars *fructose* and *galactose*. All three of these are monosaccharides, or simple sugars. Galactose is converted to glucose and metabolized through the same metabolic pathways. But fructose, as you're about to learn, is a different animal entirely. It doesn't raise blood sugar—a selling point (at least for the nutritionally naïve) for fructose-rich agave nectar. Fructose, when it's separated from the natural fibers that buffer its metabolism, destroys your liver instead.

The Fructose Story

Table sugar, or sucrose, is a disaccharide—two molecules of sugar holding hands: fructose and glucose. Lactose, the sugar in milk, is also a disaccharide: glucose and galactose. High-fructose corn syrup (HFCS) is a mixture of fructose and glucose that is most commonly 55 percent fructose and 45 percent glucose. It gets a deservedly bad rap, but it's good to recognize that table sugar contains almost the same amount of fructose as HFCS.

Fructose, or fruit sugar, is absorbed in the small intestine, and then travels through the portal vein to the liver, where almost all of it is processed. Unlike glucose, fructose is low on the glycemic index. It doesn't cause a release of insulin, which is generally touted as a good thing. But glycemic index isn't the only determinant of health. Some of the fructose enters the metabolic pathway for glycogenesis and is stored as glycogen. But the big deal about fructose is that it's highly *lipogenic*, meaning that it turns into fat in a New York minute.

The prodigious capacity of fructose to turn into fat shows up on your belly, hips, and thighs.[1] But here's the big red flag: Much of that fructose-generated fat gets stored in the liver itself, causing a bizarre condition called *nonalcoholic fatty liver disease* (NAFLD).

Developing the human equivalent of foie gras, unfortunately, is no rarity. Stop for a moment and take this in: *One-third* of Americans, including 14 percent of our precious children, have nonalcoholic fatty liver disease. It's a major cause of cirrhosis of the liver and is associated with both insulin resistance and metabolic syndrome, the two big metabolic bogeymen we'll get to shortly.

> Holy moly. You don't even have to drink to kill your liver. Well, that's not quite right. You don't have to drink alcohol. Soda or lemonade, apple juice, orange juice, or sports drinks can do the trick just as well.

Dr. Robert Lustig, M.D., a pediatric endocrinologist and highly respected authority on childhood obesity, compares soft drinks to alcohol without the buzz. You wouldn't give your young children beer, he suggests, so why would you let them drink HFCS-containing beverages?

Children don't have to chug down a Big Gulp to load up on sugar. Lustig is concerned about the epidemic of obese six-month-olds. A can of formula, he points out, is full of sugar. It's essentially a baby milkshake. Furthermore, the earlier you expose kids to sweet tastes, the more they crave it later. This is also true before birth. The more sugar a pregnant mother eats or drinks, the more her baby's fat metabolism is changed before birth. And as you'll discover when we discuss epigenetics, what a pregnant mother eats also changes her baby's *epigenome*—its genetic control panel—and thus its metabolism, sometimes for life.

You can view Lustig's famous University of California TV channel lecture "Sugar: The Bitter Truth" on YouTube at www.youtube.com/watch?v=dBnniua6-oM. His 89-minute video, which was uploaded in July of 2009, has been viewed over 4,000,000 times and counting. I think it should be required viewing for every parent, teacher, health-care professional, and politician. If you haven't watched it, I sincerely hope you will.

Some of Lustig's most salient points concern the consumption of high-fructose corn syrup. We were never exposed to the stuff before 1975. We now drink a national average of 63 pounds per person annually. That's a lot of calories, but calories aren't the main problem. The main problem is . . . that fructose is a poison. Really?

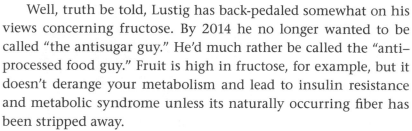

Well, truth be told, Lustig has back-pedaled somewhat on his views concerning fructose. By 2014 he no longer wanted to be called "the antisugar guy." He'd much rather be called the "anti–processed food guy." Fruit is high in fructose, for example, but it doesn't derange your metabolism and lead to insulin resistance and metabolic syndrome unless its naturally occurring fiber has been stripped away.

An interesting part of Lustig's "Sugar: The Bitter Truth" lecture is the epic story he tells about the rise of fiber-poor processed foods that began in 1973. President Nixon was concerned that rising food prices might cost him the election, so he instructed his secretary of agriculture, Earl Butz—a champion of large-scale corporate farming—to focus on providing Americans with cheap food. As it happened, high-fructose corn syrup had been invented in Japan in 1966. Lustig jokes that it was their revenge for losing World War II.

Under the influence of Butz, corn found a whole new life when, in 1975, food companies began to add HFCS to cheap processed foods to improve palatability. It's now in ketchup and bread; hamburger buns and pretzels; soda and salad dressing; chicken nuggets and breakfast cereal. In fact, HFCS is a component of almost any processed food you can name.

The Food and Nutrition Service of the Department of Agriculture under Nixon also created WIC: Women, Infants, and Children. It was and is a much-needed program. According to its website (www.fns.usda.gov/wic), "The Special Supplemental Nutrition Program for Women, Infants, and Children (WIC) provides Federal grants to States for supplemental foods, health care referrals, and nutrition education for low-income pregnant, breastfeeding, and nonbreastfeeding postpartum women, and to infants and children up to age five who are found to be at nutritional risk."

Unfortunately, one of the foods that WIC provides to poor children is fruit juice. According to Lustig, not only does the number of fruit juice servings per day predict obesity, but it also increases the risk for type 2 diabetes.

When my own kids were small, like most people I believed that fruit juice was good for them. Even though our budget was tight, we scrimped on other things to buy organic juice. Orange juice. Apple juice. Grape juice. My boys drank it for breakfast and for snacks. We froze it as a substitute for popsicles. We threw it into the blender with bananas to make what we truly believed were healthy smoothies. They loved it, of course, since juice is so sweet.

Like most parents we did the best we could for our kids. Unfortunately, we didn't know about the metabolism of fructose back then. But we do know it now, hopefully in time to stem the epidemic of childhood obesity and type 2 diabetes that's ravishing my grandchildren's generation.

Fructose is almost twice as sweet as glucose. That's another incentive for Big Food to use it. It doesn't take much to give food the oversweet taste we've become accustomed to. After a few weeks of a PlantPlus lifestyle, you'll most likely wonder how you could ever have tolerated that degree of sweetness. Unless you have a gene for a sweet tooth (yes, such a gene actually exists), the level of sweetness that the average consumer has gotten used to is just plain nasty tasting.

In 1982 the United States Department of Agriculture launched Part 3 of what Lustig considers the perfect fructose storm. They instructed us to reduce fat consumption in order to reduce heart disease. When fat is taken out of processed foods, the result is bland and tasteless. Since food companies have phenomenal laboratories run by excellent chemists charged with creating addictively tasty food, the missing fat was soon replaced by sugar.

When fat got the boot, HFCS filled the void, or at least most of the void. Salt filled the rest. If you want to read an eye-opener of a book about the food industry, written by a skilled investigative reporter, get *Salt Sugar Fat: How the Food Giants Hooked Us* by Michael Moss.

> The bottom line is that when you see the words *low fat* on any processed-food product, your only safe option is to run at top speed in the other direction.

In my grandparents' time at the turn of the 20th century, the average person consumed 15 grams (about 4 teaspoons or half an ounce) of fructose daily. This all came from fiber-rich vegetables and fruits. Today, on average, we consume four to five times that amount, children being the biggest customers. Much of that excess comes from fiber-free soft drinks and fruit juices. Without fiber there's nothing to slow the absorption of fructose into the body. And there's nothing to signal the brain that we've eaten, or to slow the absorption of free fatty acids into fat cells.

We now "mainline" fructose as well as glucose and, as a result, metabolism becomes deranged and we store more and more fat.

A Big Gulp soft drink is 55 ounces. I applaud former mayor of New York Michael Bloomberg for his efforts to outlaw soft drinks the size of wading pools. The original colas, in contrast, were only six ounces. They weren't good for you, but they had the benefit of being about a tenth the size of what a kid can buy at most gas stations and convenience stores for 99 cents.

The kid who's drinking Big Gulps is unfortunately likelier to develop hypertension as well as to get fat. Fructose is metabolized to uric acid, a molecule that blocks nitric oxide, which relaxes blood vessels and lowers blood pressure. So the more soda a child drinks, the higher their blood pressure and uric acid levels are likely to be.

What's particularly bothersome about fructose is its relationship to *insulin resistance*—a sure sign that metabolism is deranged. *Listen up, since the most important factor in choosing a diet right for your metabolic type is whether or not you are insulin resistant.*

The bottom line? Fructose is okay when it's in whole fruits and vegetables. It's added sugar—both fructose *and* glucose—that are wrecking our health and expanding the national waistline.

Get Real About How Much Sugar to Eat

In 2014 the World Health Organization halved its recommendation of the amount of sugar safe to eat, from 10 percent to 5 percent of daily calories. The average American consumes just over

22 teaspoons of sugar each day! No kidding. The recommended amount is just 5 to 6 teaspoons—20 to 24 grams (g)—for an average woman of normal weight, and about 9 teaspoons (36 g) for an average man of normal weight.

How about kids? Three teaspoons (12 g) is the recommendation. A lot of kids eat two or three times that much just for breakfast.

So let's do a get-real check of the sugar content in some common foods. Bear in mind that one teaspoon of sugar equals four grams:

- Can of soda = 10 teaspoons (40 g)
- One serving (¾ cup) Cap'n Crunch cereal = 3 teaspoons (12 g)
- Pop-Tart (chocolate fudge) = 5 teaspoons (20 g)
- Dunkin' Donuts blueberry-crumb doughnut = 13 teaspoons (52 g) (Admittedly their highest sugar variety; a chocolate-glazed doughnut is just over 3 teaspoons [13 g])
- Nature Valley Crunchy Granola Bar = 3 teaspoons (12 g)
- Jamba Juice Banana Berry smoothie (small) = 15 teaspoons (60 g)
- Ketchup (one tablespoon) = almost a teaspoon (3.4 g)
- Fruit-flavored yogurt = 6+ teaspoons (average of 26 g)
- Heinz classic tomato soup = almost 4 teaspoons (15 g)
- Panera Bread carrot cake with walnuts = 15½ teaspoons (62 g)

Become a Sugar Sleuth

Read labels religiously! Better yet, eat whole foods that have no sugar added.

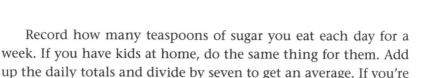

Record how many teaspoons of sugar you eat each day for a week. If you have kids at home, do the same thing for them. Add up the daily totals and divide by seven to get an average. If you're near the recommended limit, congratulations. If you're over the limit, congratulations for just doing this exercise.

Awareness is the beginning of making positive changes. For every teaspoon over the limit, try cutting back to half that amount the following week. If your child is at 20 teaspoons a day, for instance, reduce their intake to 10 teaspoons. Remember, that's the amount in a single can of soda. Ten teaspoons is still more than three times over the limit, but it's a start. The following week cut their sugar back to 5 teaspoons day. That's still almost twice the recommended amount. The following week cut them back to 3 teaspoons daily.

Make a game of reading labels and finding healthier choices. Most kids love sliced apples with peanut or almond butter, for example. But beware. Many brands of nut butter also contain added sugar. Read the label and choose a natural brand without sugar. Or bake some of my delicious low-sugar cookies that you'll find in Part IV.

It's fine to have a treat once in a while, but when once in a while means every day, you've got an addiction going. If you like doughnuts, for instance, keep them to once a week. If your kids like dry cereal, check the labels. Some cereals have as little as a gram of added sugar per serving. Others are the same or even worse than eating a candy bar.

Make a game out of being healthy, and ask your kids—if you have any—to play it with you.

In Chapter 23, there's a list of ingredients that are synonyms for sugar—rapadura or brown-rice syrup, for example. Can you find the hidden sugar when you read down a list of ingredients?

Even if you're a normal weight, don't get complacent. You may be thin on the outside, but fat on the inside (TOFI). That means that you've got fat around your internal organs. TOFI folks are likely to develop metabolic syndrome, the consummate health villain that leads to diabetes, heart disease, and neurological problems.

Metabolic syndrome and insulin resistance are the meanest gunslingers in the OK Corral. You'll learn all about why that is in the next healthful, ultralow-sugar Science Bite.

CHAPTER 9

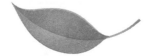

Help! I'm Fat and I'm Famished:

Insulin Resistance and Metabolic Syndrome

"The two biggest sellers in bookstores are the cookbooks and the diet books. The cookbooks tell you how to prepare the food and the diet books tell you how not to eat any of it."

— ANDY ROONEY

Bob, a man in his 40s, was a participant in a workshop I was giving on the new brain science. When he heard that I was writing a book on personalized nutrition, he cornered me in the hallway desperate for some advice. "Help," he said in exasperation, shifting from one foot to the other, and then taking a deep breath and meeting my eyes. "I'm fat, but I'm famished. What's going on with that? It just doesn't seem right."

It isn't right, but it sure is common. The epidemic of obesity is so out of hand that 70 percent of Americans are in the same boat that Bob is. They've got weight around the middle, have trouble losing it, and often—though they may not know it—suffer from insulin resistance. That means that their cells aren't too quick to answer the doorbell when insulin comes calling. Instead, it gets left standing outside with a bag full of sugar.

The pancreatic beta cells that manufacture and ship the insulin out still work fine. But the exquisitely sensitive dance between the insulin molecule and its receptor turns clumsy and out of sync. Blood sugar rises and begins to create a cascade of metabolic anomalies that increase the risk for type 2 diabetes; double the risk of heart disease; and predispose people like Bob to stroke, osteoporosis, and the entire lineup of "your ticket is almost expired" diseases.

Glucose on the loose, freed to create advanced glycation end products, or AGEs, eventually damages the eyes, nerves, kidneys, and heart. Fortunately, insulin resistance and metabolic syndrome can be reduced or reversed by losing weight.

Gotcha! That's the catch-22. How can you lose weight if you're always hungry? Let's take a look at metabolic syndrome first; then we'll turn our attention to the Fat-Storage Trifecta—the three factors that contribute to being fat and famished.

Metabolic Syndrome

Although insulin resistance is a major factor in the development of metabolic syndrome, there may be other factors involved as well: genetics, sitting too long at one stretch, different species of gut bacteria, and the epigenetic effects of stress and the foods we eat. The National Heart, Lung, and Blood Institute (NHLBI) as well as the American Heart Association (AHA) recommend a diagnosis of metabolic syndrome if you've got three or more of the following conditions.[1]

1. An apple shape. You qualify as an apple if you've got some belly fat happening—if you're a woman with a waist circumference of 35 inches or greater or a man whose waist is more than 40 inches around. Belly fat isn't a dusty old storage locker either. It's a metabolically active factory that churns out inflammatory hormones as well as the appetite-suppressant hormone *leptin*. If you become insulin resistant, then leptin resistance follows, so hunger ramps up. Your fat cells don't get the message that they're already full, so of course you want to eat more often. A Buddha belly also churns out dangerous immune factors called *pro-inflammatory cytokines* that create the low-level inflammation that underlies heart disease, osteoporosis, and virtually any other chronic condition you can think of.

The hormones and immune factors that belly fat releases travel to the liver via the portal vein where they wreak havoc with the production of blood lipids like triglycerides and cholesterol, causing what's called *dyslipidemia*, the dangerous set of changes in triglycerides and cholesterol that you'll read about next.

2. High triglyceride levels of more than 150 mg/dl (milligrams per deciliter). Triglycerides, or blood fat, are made by the liver and then shipped out in lipoprotein "trucks" or particles that deliver the goods to muscle and fat cells. When you become insulin resistant, too many triglycerides get manufactured and shipped out, a risk factor for heart disease and stroke.

3. Low HDL cholesterol (the "good" cholesterol). Levels less than 40 mg/dl for men and less than 50 mg/dl for women are considered low and are a risk factor for heart disease. Ideally your HDLs ought to be 60 mg/dl or higher.

4. High blood pressure of 130/85 mm Hg (millimeters of mercury) or higher (although at this writing, docs are arguing vociferously about new guidelines). Normal blood pressure, at least until recently, was defined as 120 mm Hg or lower for systolic pressure (the top number), and 80 mm Hg or lower for diastolic pressure (the bottom number).

5. Elevated fasting blood glucose equal to or greater than 100 mg/dl. Uh oh, if you're hyperglycemic that means that the AGEing process is on. Your insides are gumming up and you're on the fast track for developing type 2 diabetes or a neurodegenerative disease.

Stop for a moment and read through this list again. Ring any bells?

If you haven't had your lipids tested lately and don't know what these numbers are, beware. Ignorance is *not* bliss. It's shocking how fast you can go from what appears to be "normal" to realizing that you have a potentially life-threatening condition like heart disease. In Chapter 18 you'll learn what tests to ask for to check up on your metabolism and determine how insulin sensitive or insulin resistant you are, and exactly what needs improvement. Having the tests done also provides a baseline for comparison after your four-week PlantPlus Reboot.

Being overweight with a diagnosis of metabolic syndrome already tells you that a low-carb diet, at least initially, is your best bet for losing weight and normalizing your metabolism. Trying to eat a high-carb diet, even if you limit portion size, is hard to pull off because *leptin resistance* makes you hungry.

Leptin Resistance

Leptin, as you know, is a hormone manufactured by fat cells. It's the "lay off the food, we're full now" hormone. If your cells become resistant to leptin, you feel hungry even if your fat cells are full. That causes the Hungry Ghost Syndrome—never feeling satisfied, at least for long.

Leptin is released into the bloodstream and travels to the hypothalamus of the brain where it turns off the urge to eat. The more overweight a person is, the larger their fat cells are, and the more leptin they make. You'd think all that leptin would make you lose interest in eating, but the opposite is true. You want to eat more!

> The more weight you gain, the more leptin resistant you're likely to become. The signal that was once a bull-horn (*stop eating!*) becomes attenuated to a soft whisper.

So what's the problem? While the mechanisms causing leptin resistance are still an active area of study, some researchers hypothesize that it might be related to an inability to metabolize cereal grains properly.[2] That's an interesting hypothesis.

In the meantime, think about how you respond to a high-carb meal. How long does it keep you satisfied? For instance, the kind of high-carb breakfast we ate as ultra-low-fat vegans—sprouted whole-grain bread with jam, and oatmeal with maple syrup and fruit—used to leave me starved after an hour. That's the result of eating more carbs than your body can efficiently process. And as the weight began to pile up, I became hungrier and hungrier, probably the beginnings of leptin resistance. Since most of the carbs we were eating came from grain, however, there's a good chance that the high concentration of lectins I was consuming were adding to the growing hunger.

The Fat-Storage Trifecta

How might a diet rich in grains contribute to metabolic problems and fat storage above and beyond adding a lot of carbs and calories to your diet? Here's a three-prong scenario for weight gain and hunger that you don't hear much about:

1. *Hyperglycemia.* Eating carbs, especially sugar and flour, floods your body with sugar. It doesn't matter whether you're eating whole-wheat, gluten-free, or white flour. Flours aren't whole grains. They're powders with a lot of surface area, easy to process into sugar. Remember, *two pieces of supposedly healthy*

whole-wheat bread are quickly metabolized into two tablespoons of sugar. The sudden rise in blood sugar turns on the body's fat-storing program.

2. *Lectins.* Lectins bind to the membranes of your cells and act like hormones that *mimic the effects of insulin.* These impostor molecules bind to a sugar molecule on the insulin receptor and initiate the program that commands, "Get busy storing fat!"

3. *Leptin insensitivity.* Lectins either block the leptin receptors or interfere with signaling to the hypothalamus in some other way that still awaits discovery. Leptin insensitivity means that although you've just stored fat, you still feel hungry. So, of course, even if you want to lose weight, you feel compelled to eat a little more. And store some more fat. And eat a little more. And store more fat. And the beat goes on.

> The Fat-Storage Trifecta is a physiological reality. The fat-storing program isn't initiated because of a lack of willpower. I really want to emphasize that. Even if you've failed at many other diets, a PlantPlus Diet that regulates carb intake and provides sufficient protein and good fat will keep you feeling full—especially if you cut out lectin-containing grains. Your problem is *not* a lack of willpower; it's all about eating the wrong foods for your metabolism.

If you're worried that you won't be able to break the grain habit, believe me, it's not as hard as you think. By eating nutrient-rich plants (they have good carbs that break down slowly and are absorbed slowly as well because of the fiber that comes with them), coupled with protein and good fats, your leptin resistance

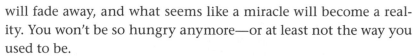

will fade away, and what seems like a miracle will become a reality. You won't be so hungry anymore—or at least not the way you used to be.

How many carbs and what kind should you be eating? That depends on what's carb-reasonable for your metabolism, a subject we'll come back to in Chapter 18 when we discuss the tests your doc can order to determine how insulin sensitive or insulin resistant you are.

Carbs and grains aren't the only factor determining insulin sensitivity, though. Exercise levels, the epigenetic effects of foods you eat, and your genome itself add to individual differences. A new field called nutrigenomics is actively exploring how these unique differences affect not only what you should be eating but also your eating behaviors.

But before we take a look at how your genes affect how you fit into your jeans, we need to investigate just how reliable scientific studies are. These days science is the new god. Both scientists and the media—as well as most laypeople—often misinterpret the results of studies or blow them all out of proportion.

No wonder nutrition is such a confusing subject.

CHAPTER 10

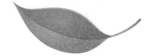

How Scientific
Is Science?

*"If we knew what it was we were doing,
it would not be called research, would it?"*

— ALBERT EINSTEIN

How trustworthy is the science we bet our lives on? As you know, the national War on Fat didn't turn out so well except if you happen to be a junk-food or pharmaceutical manufacturer. Unfortunately, most studies in medical journals (not just nutrition studies) don't pass muster with skilled statisticians. Much of the data analysis is plain old wrong, which doesn't stop sketchy results from becoming the Holy Grail of what's called "evidence-based" medical practice.

That's an eye-opener, since many of us—including the media—assume reflexively that any peer-reviewed medical study published in a prestigious journal is reliable. We also tend to accept research and anecdotes that confirm our prejudices while ignoring or rejecting research that challenges or refutes deeply held beliefs. Emotions can and do easily trump reason. And make no mistake. Food is a highly charged and emotional topic.

Thus . . .

Meat eaters can find plenty of studies that report no difference in longevity between omnivores and vegetarians.

Vegetarians can likewise cite studies concluding that vegetarians live longer, healthier lives than omnivores.

Vegans and raw foodists refuting their previous lifestyle often cite data showing that veganism is harmful to your health, or at least likely to make your teeth fall out.

Devotees of ancestral diets base their food choices on ethnographic records revealing that in Paleolithic times we ate diets rich in meat and whatever vegetation we could forage for. Only when agriculture came into the picture in Neolithic times did we begin to cultivate grains, which were not genetically suited to our metabolism.

Adherents of nutrient-rich, low-calorie plant-based diets remind us that we share 98 percent to 99 percent of our genes with chimps and baboons and therefore should subsist mostly on leaves, fruits, and perhaps the equivalent of a few grubs or flying squirrels.

So it's no wonder that most people, including physicians, can't make heads nor tails of what we're best off eating and why. Most people I talk to about diet tell me that they're confused.

Woody Allen poked fun at our society's perpetual food quandary and quest for health in his futuristic 1973 film, *Sleeper*. There's a prescient scene in which his character has just awakened in the future from a 200-year cryogenic sleep. One of his physicians chuckles when Allen asks for wheat germ, organic honey, and Tiger's Milk—foods thought to be healthful a couple of centuries earlier. Hot fudge and "deep fat" are the health foods of the fictional future. Sometimes art really does imitate life.

So how do we actually know whether what we choose to eat is healthy or not? Since we're a society that believes in science with a zeal that rivals religious fanaticism, it's important to ponder the question of how accurate scientific studies actually are.

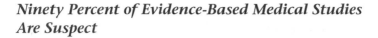

Ninety Percent of Evidence-Based Medical Studies Are Suspect

One of the most popular medical speakers in the world is a Harvard-trained physician and consummate statistician by the name of John Ioannidis, M.D. Journalist David Freedman wrote an excellent article about him in *The Atlantic* magazine in 2012 entitled "Lies, Damned Lies, and Medical Science."

He wrote that Ioannidis and his colleagues "have shown, again and again, and in many different ways, that much of what bio-medical researchers conclude in published studies—conclusions that doctors keep in mind when they prescribe antibiotics or blood-pressure medication, or when they advise us to consume more fiber or less meat, or when they recommend surgery for heart disease or back pain—is misleading, exaggerated, and often flat-out wrong."[1] He charges that as much as 90 percent of the published medical information that doctors rely on is flawed.

Good grief. This is a very inconvenient truth to say the least.

> Fifty-plus years of science, which is now either disproven or in question, told us that fat was our mortal enemy. As a result of following recommendations to lower fat intake, we are now a nation that is both fat and sick.

After you've finished reading this chapter, you'll know a lot about why that's so.

Our Love Affair with Anecdotes

When someone tells you that a particular diet cured their cancer, restored their fertility, or made them thin and sexy, it's appropriate to congratulate them. It's not appropriate to base your own diet on their anecdotal experience. Unfortunately, many people do just that. "Well, eating this or that cured him or her, so I'll eat it, too."

Maybe it cured them or maybe it didn't, but anecdotes do not science make. Just the belief that something will cure you or make you better produces a positive result about 50 percent of the time. This is called the *placebo effect,* and it's the bane of researchers and drug companies. It's also a fascinating mind-body phenomenon.

Recent research, in fact, has shown that almost all the benefit reported from antidepressant drugs is due to the placebo effect. Older research highlighted the results of sham surgery for knee pain. In the placebo group an incision was made and sutured up, but nothing was changed in the knee joint. It's wonderful that some of the people who received the sham surgery could play basketball again, but the result was due to their faith in the surgery rather than a change in their anatomy.

> *Anecdotes are not research studies.* They're case reports. Their only value (other than to the person who got great results) is to generate a scientific hypothesis that can then be tested in a real study, preferably a *randomized controlled double-blind study.*

Randomized controlled double-blind studies are the Rolls Royce of study design. Research subjects are randomly assigned to either a placebo treatment or a potentially active treatment. *Double-blind* means that neither the researcher nor the research subject know which group they've been assigned to. In this way, the important and powerful effects of belief are controlled. This type of study is the likeliest to generate data that can be trusted, but there are still a lot of slips between the cup and the lip.

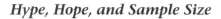

Hype, Hope, and Sample Size

When you get wind of a study being hyped by the media, something like "Eating an egg is as bad as smoking a cigarette" or "Eating meat in middle age causes cancer," take a deep breath and put on your thinking cap.

Was the study large or small? Who is the first author? A vegan who does a study on the evils of meat is likely to reach different conclusions than an omnivore might. And when a company that trades in grains funds a study, the results are significantly more likely to support their products than not. Ditto for the dairy industry and other special-interest groups.

Then there's the matter of sample size. How many people need to be studied in order to generate statistically valid conclusions? When I was still a research scientist, I wanted to design a study that compared physical symptoms, psychological state, quality of life, and length of survival in cancer patients who got usual treatment plus a "placebo" support group to patients who got usual treatment plus instructions in meditation, self-regulation, and finding meaning as well as support. Given our resources, the study wasn't feasible because we would have needed thousands of volunteers to control for all the different variables and come out with meaningful results.

Leaving Out Crucial Facts

The research that you hear about in the news is often so watered down that essential facts go missing and the public is left with an erroneous conclusion. Here's a case in point. A 2013 study published in the journal *Nature Medicine*[2] involved a substance called TMAO, which is made when a certain species of bacteria ferments carnitine (found in red meat, fish, peas, carrots, and a variety of other foods including energy drinks) into a gas that passes through the wall of the gut into the bloodstream.

Mice whose drinking water was supplemented with carnitine developed twice the amount of plaque in their arteries as a control group who didn't get any carnitine. Another part of the experiment involved feeding eight-ounce steaks plus a carnitine pill to five omnivores and one brave vegan. The vegan didn't ferment the carnitine to TMAO. This study was widely hyped by the media as proof that eating red meat causes cardiovascular disease.

Here are a few of the problems with the study. First, the fact that some vegetables and fish contain as much or more carnitine than red meat wasn't mentioned. Second, a study of one vegan isn't a study—it's one case and has no statistical power. I'll let a brilliant microbiologist, Jeff Leach, tell you about another problem, one of many that he explains with clarity in his blog post, "From Meat to Microbes to Main Street: Is It Time to Trade In Your George Foreman Grill?"

Leach is one of the world's foremost authorities on gut microbes and their anthropological distribution. With colleagues at the University of Colorado in Boulder and the Argonne National Laboratory, he launched a very large-scale, crowd-funded citizen science initiative that's documenting the microbial ecosystem in the guts of 10,000 American volunteers.

Leach wrote the following about how the media reported the TMAO study:

> Most failed to mention the mice used in the study (Apoe -/- mice) are genetically engineered to be prone to atherosclerosis. On top of that, the 1.3 percent of carnitine in the drinking water is the equivalent to a human eating ~1,000 steaks a day. You can decide for yourself if you think mice that are genetically engineered to be inclined to atherosclerosis that are fed the human equivalent of an entire cow every three days for 10 weeks is proof that carnitine from red meat accelerates atherosclerosis in humans.[3]

When the TMAO study came out, I went to the Internet to:

1. Read the study and make as much sense of it as I could.

2. Check expert sites and see what some of the folks in the know had to say. Admittedly, there is generally

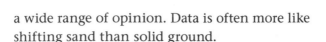

a wide range of opinion. Data is often more like shifting sand than solid ground.

Of Mice and Men

Another problem with vetting research comes from extending the results of animal studies to human beings. A 2013 study out of the University of Michigan, for example, conducted by a prestigious group of neuroscientists and published in the equally prestigious *Proceedings of the National Academy of Science,* involved euthanizing rats while measuring their brain activity. A large burst of brain activity just after death was bandied about in the media as an explanation for human near-death experiences.[4]

That's comparing apples to oranges, to put it mildly . . . and politely. To put it more realistically, such a conclusion—or even allusion—is patently ridiculous. Some animal studies, of course, are more relevant to humans than others. A study of wound healing, for example, is more pertinent to human biology than a study involving consciousness. Studies of metabolism and gut microbes in rodents or rabbits can also yield preliminary hypotheses that can then be tested in human beings.

But with few exceptions, it's important to realize that most people aren't rats.

The Red Herring Effect

Observational studies mine data from large cohorts of people like nurses, people who get their care at the same HMO for years, or people who live in a specific geographical area, to name just a few examples. Data from the cohort might include medical tests, psychological questionnaires, or self-reports about mood, food, social support, or what have you. There may be data about what people claim to eat, the quality of their sleep, whether they pray, how much exercise they get, or the geographical area they hail from.

Researchers comb through the records years later, comparing the data on hand to recent health records or death certificates. Observational studies ask questions like, Do omnivores develop more heart disease than vegetarians? Do people with high cholesterol have more heart attacks? Do people who eat lots of greens have fewer strokes? Do joyful people live longer than sad sacks?

In this era of sparse research funding, when the academic ethos is still "publish or perish," observational studies are popular because they're relatively cheap, easy to do, and translate into publishing more papers over time and thus keeping your job.

> The big problem is that *observational studies cannot establish causation*. They can only report correlations. For example, just because people with diabetes have twice the rate of Alzheimer's disease as those who don't, you can't conclude that diabetes causes Alzheimer's disease. It's imperative to look for the underlying mechanism that increases the incidence of both ailments.

Let me give you an example of an observational study that caused a big stir. Women on hormone replacement therapy (HRT) were reported to have less heart disease. When word of this correlation got out, it was, unfortunately, treated like a causal relationship. Women beat a path to their doctors' doors in order to get prescriptions for HRT to protect their hearts.

An obvious explanation for the correlation between HRT and heart health might have been that health-conscious women were more likely to ask their docs for HRT than women who weren't as proactive. Their healthy lifestyle, rather than the hormones, could have produced the correlation. And indeed, that's exactly what happened. When better-designed studies showed that HRT can actually *cause* heart disease, the sound of women gasping could be heard throughout the land.

Observational studies can generate hypotheses for testing in more scientifically rigorous, prospective, randomized, double-blind studies. In the latter type of study, as you know from our previous discussion, there's both a control group and an experimental group who start out healthy and are then followed over time. That's what *prospective* means.

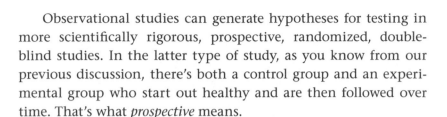

Only a prospective study can make claims about causation—for instance, that exercise actually reduces depression or that an apple a day might keep the doctor away.

Same Study, Different Results, Anyone?

Let me quote from a paper based on a meta-analysis, a study of studies that looks at pooled data, investigating whether omega-3 fatty acids (scientists refer to these as n-3 PUFA) reduce the rate of breast cancer in women. A 2013 paper published in the *British Medical Journal* illustrates just how confusing nutritional science can be—even in the case of prospective studies:

> Results from observational studies in humans, however, are inconsistent. . . . Prospective studies suggest that fish, the richest source of marine n-3 PUFA, shows inverse, null, or even positive associations with risk.[5]

The kind of quote you just read about n-3 PUFAs—essentially saying that we don't really know which end is up—is not unusual. Scientists, even in the same laboratory, can repeat the same experiment and get different results. A good rule of thumb is to repeat a study at least three times and see if the data can be replicated. If not, it's time to go back to the drawing board. But because studies can be massively expensive to do and very time-consuming—think years—it's hard or even impossible for scientists always to replicate their results.

Thus, the common statement that follows almost all research announcements: "More studies are needed."

The Single-Nutrient Dilemma

Another problem with nutritional studies concerns the dubious undertaking of isolating *single nutrients* from food and then making health claims about them. Citrus fruits have a lot of vitamin C, for instance, but they have thousands of other micronutrients as well. Some of those micronutrients are, of course, synergistic with one another.

Basing conclusions on single-nutrient data has been compared to moving one piece in a Rubik's Cube without recognizing that all the pieces around it will also move. For example, vitamin E is a powerful antioxidant. But given as a supplement, or in multivitamins, there's data that it shortens the human life span. The apparent reason for that is that in high doses, isolated from the foods that naturally contain it, vitamin E inhibits some of the body's innate antioxidant systems.

I'm often asked my opinion about vitamins and supplements. Since I'm wary of taking nutrients out of their natural context, I err on the side of caution. What if one day's miracle supplement turns out to be the next decade's deadly debacle?

On the other hand, sometimes a deficiency in a particular micronutrient really does need to be remediated. For example, if a pregnant mom is folate deficient, neural-tube defects like spina bifida can occur in the fetus. So it's a good idea to consult your physician about what vitamins or other supplements may be right for you. Is he or she right? Who knows. That's why it's good to check as many other expert opinions as possible, photocopy what you find, and discuss it with your doctor.

Some of my go-to sites for information about nutrition are www.theeatingacademy.com, www.drweil.com, www.chriskresser.com, and www.humanfoodproject.com. Because these sites are so different, they yield a spectrum of opinion and expertise. A recent blog post by Peter Attia, M.D., on his very cool and informative site (www.theeatingacademy.com) is a case in point about what to believe and whose opinions are worth checking.

In his blog, Dr. Attia was discussing the evolution of his diet, specifically that he was craving more vegetables and less meat.

He anticipated the following question: Did he cut down on meat based on his body's own personal needs, or was his decision based on studies on the putative negative effects of eating red meat? Here's part of his blog post:

> Because I know someone will ask—do I think red meat is harmful?—the answer is no, I do not believe so. Certainly not based on evidence I've seen to date, including the recent story about protein. For those looking to brush up on the state of evidence implicating red meat, I'd recommend three posts—one I wrote many moons ago in response to one of the dozen epidemiology stories, one written by Chris Masterjohn in response to the TMAO data, and one recently by Zoe Harcombe in response to the protein epidemiology.[6]

Even experts turn to other experts for help in thinking through the flood of research that rains down upon us daily.

That said, let's turn our attention back to you. With the Plant-Plus Diet, you get to be your own lab rat. One person does not a study make, but if you base your food choices on the best available scientific hypotheses, and then track observable changes in your medical tests and your Medical Symptom Checklist, you can become an effective researcher in regard to your *own* health.

Ready. Set. Go. Let the sleuthing begin.

CHAPTER 11

Personalized Metabolism:
The A to Z Study

*"It's less a matter of crowning a single winning diet than of
finding the winning match between a diet and an individual."*

— CHRISTOPHER GARDNER

Christopher Gardner, Ph.D., a longtime vegetarian, is also the
director of nutrition studies at the Stanford Prevention Research
Center. Although he's been a vegetarian for many years—in fact,
he decided to study nutrition in the first place so that his friends
wouldn't make fun of him—he seems honestly open and without bias when it comes down to what a particular person is best
off eating. Dr. Gardner is a scientist interested in how we can go
about reversing the epidemic of obesity that's bankrupting our
nation and creating so much personal misery, whatever that takes
for each one of us.

But unless you tried every one of the major diet types—from
Atkins to Zone—in a methodical way (what Gardner did in a series of research studies), how would you know which diet worked
best for you? A look at Gardner's original study, and a follow-up

study that looked at the effect of genotype on diet effectiveness, provides some clues about how to match diet to metabolic type.

The A TO Z Study

Gardner's original 2007 study was called the A TO Z Study.[1] It was published in the prestigious *Journal of the American Medical Association* (*JAMA*). While that distinction doesn't always equate to good science, the A TO Z Study does. It was landmark research for several reasons.

First of all, it compared three popular diets ranging in carbohydrate and fat content with "usual" nutritional care—typical government dietary recommendations. *A* stands for Atkins (very low carb, high fat); *T* stands for traditional, based on the low-fat, high-carb government food pyramid with instructions on portion control (a Yale program called LEARN); *O* stands for Ornish (very low fat, high carb); and *Z* stands for Zone (intermediate carb).

Second, it studied 311 overweight or obese women, a sufficient number of research subjects to generate statistical power, meaning that chance results based on small sample size were less likely.

Third, the study lasted for a year. That's important since many diet studies last for only a few months. That's not long enough to see how many people can stick to the diet and either lose weight or improve health markers over a longer time period.

Fourth, it had relatively few dropouts. That's very important since, generally speaking, people in a diet study who don't lose weight feel bad about it and don't come back. They might feel embarrassed, be concerned about ruining the study, or both. In fact, a high dropout rate often does compromise or even ruin a study.

As a long-term vegetarian, Dr. Gardner was originally betting on the near-vegan Ornish program as the diet that would be the healthiest and most effective in terms of weight loss. As he said in an interview with low-carb blogger Jimmy Moore in 2012, he had consumed "the low-fat Koolaid."

It was a surprise to Gardner when the group that lost the most weight in the A TO Z Study was, in fact, the very-low-carb, high-fat

Atkins group. They also had the greatest improvement in their lipid profiles and other metabolic markers. It was, Gardner admitted jokingly, a bitter pill for a near vegan to swallow.

Another strong point of Gardner's research is that the participants were asked to study one-eighth of a popular book about the diet they had been assigned to before each of eight weekly group sessions. During the session a very enthusiastic nutritionist would go over the content with the participants to make sure they really understood, and could implement, what they'd read. This means that the study results are relevant to anyone who is willing to read a diet book carefully and follow the program.

In a follow-up study, Gardner and his associates looked at adherence to the diets. They divided the women in each group into tertiles (thirds) and compared the most adherent third of each group with the least adherent third. The most adherent lost considerable weight, whereas the least adherent lost little or nothing. Some even gained weight.

So Who Were the Big Losers?

Atkins and Ornish were the easiest diets to adhere to because they had no calorie restrictions and the point of each was quite clear. Reduce fat for Ornish and carbs for Atkins. Zone and LEARN on the other hand had a lot of detailed instructions, calorie limits, and counting involved. They were more confusing and harder to stick with.

The most fascinating part of the study—the part that's really interesting in terms of matching a person to the right diet for their metabolic type—is that within each group there was considerable variation in the amount of weight the women lost. Some lost up to 40 pounds in a year. Others lost nothing.

So who were the big losers? *Insulin resistance turned out to be the key.*

Insulin resistance is a prediabetic state. When the body is presented with carbs, the pancreas of an insulin-resistant person keeps cranking out more and more insulin, but their cells have become relatively insensitive to it. As a result, blood glucose rises, AGEs accumulate, inflammation increases, and metabolic syndrome and diabetes soon follow.

There was a gradation of insulin resistance among women in each study group. So once again, Gardner and his associates separated the participant data into tertiles (thirds). They ignored those in the middle tertile and compared the extremes at either end of the spectrum. *The most insulin-resistant women did worst on the Ornish low-fat, high-carb diet.* If you're intrigued, take an hour to watch Dr. Gardner's informative (and very engaging) video about the study.[2] He's a cool guy who makes science fun and accessible.

> If you're insulin resistant, there's no point loading up on carbs, which the body is unable to process normally. That makes perfect sense, yes?

The Atkins Diet, on the other hand, eliminates most carbs, reducing insulin levels so that fat can be burned.

> Insulin is the fat-storage hormone. So if you need to lose weight, you also need to reduce circulating insulin levels. When insulin levels drop to more normal levels, so does weight. That alone has a spectacular effect on health. Even modest weight losses often lead to significant improvements in metabolic measures, blood pressure, type 2 diabetes, and general health.

Testing Your Insulin Resistance

Fortunately, there's a simple, relatively inexpensive blood test that can give you and your doctor the information you need . . . a score ranging from 0 to 100 rating your insulin resistance. We'll go through the specific tests you need to personalize your diet shortly. But even without a composite test score for insulin resistance, your fasting blood glucose and insulin levels can help you decide which type of diet is most likely to work for you.

The more overweight you are, the more insulin resistant you're likely to be. But there's still a range among people. If you're insulin sensitive, according to Gardner, it doesn't make much difference what diet you choose in terms of weight loss. But if you meet the criteria for metabolic syndrome, a high-carb diet is the least likely to be a good choice.

Gardner explained to Jimmy Moore that the national "low-fat mantra" is actually contributing to obesity as it predisposes insulin-resistant folks to gaining weight since the base of our food pyramid is carbohydrates, often the high-glycemic-index kind found in flour and especially in processed foods. Twenty or 30 years ago, Gardner commented, eating a diet based on carbs wasn't so much of a problem since fewer people were obese and insulin resistant. Now a low-fat diet is wrong for a larger and larger part of the population.

Once a person has lost weight, the composition of the three macronutrients in their diet—fats, carbs, and proteins—also has a lot to do with keeping that weight off. Studies show that only one in six overweight people will maintain even 10 percent of their weight loss over the long haul. That's depressing.

So why is that the case? There are two hypotheses. The first is that over time it just gets too hard to stick to the diet. People feel deprived and long for the "good" old days of eating what they like. Little by little the old ways creep back in and lead to a weight gain comparable to and even greater than in the old days. Second, after people lose weight, they don't burn as many calories. This means that they need to eat less because their body mass is smaller and they aren't using as much energy.

The big question of how we maintain our dietary gains (in this case, losses) requires us to look at the dogma that a calorie is a calorie and appreciate why that dogma is now dead. That's the subject of the next chapter.

CHAPTER 12

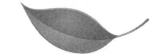

The Fat and Calorie War

"The point to keep in mind is that you don't lose fat because you cut calories; you lose fat because you cut out the foods that make you fat—the carbohydrates."

— GARY TAUBES, *WHY WE GET FAT: AND WHAT TO DO ABOUT IT*

Cara Ebbeling, Ph.D., associate director of the New Balance Foundation Obesity Prevention Center at Boston Children's Hospital, decided to look at the effects of diet *composition* on energy expenditure. She and her colleagues, including the director of the Center, David Ludwig, M.D., tested three different diets that varied in carb levels to see how they affected how many calories their experimental subjects burned.

First they put 21 overweight and obese young adults on a supervised diet so that they lost 10 to 15 percent of their body weight. The 21 subjects were then rotated through three different diets, in random order, for four weeks each: a low-fat, high-carb diet; a low-glycemic-index diet with moderate carb and fat levels; and a very-low-carb, high-fat diet.

Folks on the low-fat diet had the lowest energy expenditure. In other words, they burned fewer calories. The ones on a low-glycemic-index diet used an intermediate level of energy. Those on a low-carb diet had the highest energy expenditure.

> The diet dogma that a calorie is a calorie no matter where it comes from is dead wrong. A calorie is definitely, absolutely, and beyond doubt not a calorie. The lower the carb content of the diet in Ebbeling's study, the more calories were burned—even though all three diet types contained the exact same number of calories.[1]

Ebbeling's small but tantalizing study, like Gardner's, was published in *JAMA*. While Gardner had a lot of research subjects, Ebbeling had relatively few. As you already know—statistical maven that you are—the Ebbeling study needs to be repeated with more subjects. Nonetheless, her results suggest that diets that reduce the surge in blood sugar after a meal—either because the food is low on the glycemic index or very low in carbs—may be more effective than a low-fat diet for lasting weight loss.

In an article in *Science Daily* that discussed the results of the Ebbeling study, Ludwig—also director of the Optimal Weight for Life Clinic at Boston's Children's Hospital—was quoted as saying, "We've found that, contrary to nutritional dogma, all calories are not created equal. Total calories burned plummeted by 300 calories on the low-fat diet compared to the low-carb diet, which would equal the number of calories typically burned in an hour of moderate-intensity physical activity."[2]

Leptin, as you may recall, is the appetite-control hormone. Not surprisingly, serum leptin was lowest in the low-fat dieters, highest in the low-carb dieters, and intermediate in the low-glycemic-index dieters. The low-fat diet was also the biggest loser—meaning that it was the least effective—when it came to insulin sensitivity.

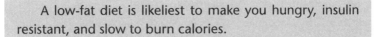

> A low-fat diet is likeliest to make you hungry, insulin resistant, and slow to burn calories.

The benefits of the low-glycemic-index diet was twofold:

1. Lower cortisol levels than the low-carb diet (higher levels can be a risk factor for heart disease)

2. Lower C-reactive protein levels, an inflammatory molecule that's also a risk factor for heart disease

This last point raised the ire of the Paleo community in the blogosphere since the meat consumed in the study was, they assume, factory farmed rather than pasture raised. That brings up an important point about diet studies. The way the food is sourced may well be critical to the outcome of the study. Eating foods containing bad fats is quite different from eating foods containing good fats.

But back to the study as it was done. Ebbeling and her co-authors concluded that the low-glycemic-index diet had the greatest overall benefit even though the low-carb diet was better at reducing markers of metabolic syndrome like low HDL and high triglycerides.

Science Daily quoted Ebbeling as saying, "In addition to the benefits noted in this study, we believe that low-glycemic-index diets are easier to stick to on a day-to-day basis, compared to low-carb and low-fat diets, which many people find limiting. Unlike low-fat and very-low-carbohydrate diets, a low-glycemic-index diet doesn't eliminate entire classes of food, likely making it easier to follow and more sustainable."

If you recall, that's not what Gardner found in his research. He claims that it's easier for most people to follow a diet that is either low in carbs or low in fat because what to eat is clear as a bell in either case.

Bottom line. The Ebbeling study needs to be replicated with a larger number of people, and also specify the foods fed to each group *and* how they were sourced. Factory-farmed meat may well create inflammation since it's adulterated with hormones, antibiotics, and pesticide residues. Since the animals are fed grain, a food that is not optimized to their metabolism, the composition of their fat also changes. It becomes higher in inflammatory omega-6 fatty acids. Pasture-raised meat, on the other hand, has more healthful anti-inflammatory omega-3 fatty acids. It's also free from hormones, pesticide residues, antibiotics, and the stress hormones that accumulate in animals who are crowded together.

Since other studies of low-carb diets have shown a decrease in inflammation, rather than the increase that the Ebbeling study reported, once again you need to be your own lab rat. If you get your C-reactive protein measured along with your insulin resistance before going on any diet plan, then you'll have a solid baseline to refer back to. That will help you decide how the composition of your diet in terms of the three macronutrients—carbs, fats, and proteins—might best be tweaked.

CHAPTER 13

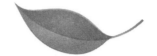

Nutrigenomics:

Matching Your Genes to Your Diet

"To the question of whether sharing 96 percent of
our genetic make-up with chimps makes us 96 percent chimp;
we also share about 50 percent of our DNA with bananas
—that does not make us half bananas!"

— Professor Steve Jones, evolutionary geneticist

Let's say that you and your best friend (or spouse) decide to go on a low-fat diet together. You eat exactly the same thing, but one of you loses a substantial amount of weight and the other one loses nary a pound. What gives with that?

It may be that you've got different genotypes.

Interleukin Genetics, Inc., in Waltham, Massachusetts, is one of several commercial genotyping companies that offer genetic testing for nutritional optimization. They've chosen the most robust (think best research design) studies of genetic differences predisposing to obesity, including what are called single nucleotide polymorphisms—SNPs (pronounced "snips")—to help people find the best diet for their genotype.

Interleukin Genetics approached Dr. Christopher Gardner about screening the saliva of women from the A TO Z Study in order to see whether those women whose genotype matched the diet they'd been given lost more weight than women whose genotype and diet weren't such a good match.

According to a synopsis of the study design registered with www.clinicaltrials.gov within the National Institutes of Health:

> Interleukin Genetics will obtain DNA samples from the previously enrolled study subjects to investigate genetic influence of the response to macronutrient compositions of low caloric diets to weight loss. . . . Interleukin Genetics has derived, through an extensive search of the scientific literature, a genetic test panel in the area of Weight Management (WM), which includes the genes that have been shown to affect body weight. These genes have been associated with elevated risk for obesity.[1]

Before we continue, dear reader, moderate your excitement—at least for now.

> Genotyping and nutrition is still an itty-bitty baby science, inexact to say the least since there are a huge number of genotypic variations that can affect metabolism. They're essentially endless, and it's going to take a tremendous amount of work to narrow them down so that genetic testing for weight loss and metabolism can become more reliable.

Nonetheless, Gardner and his colleagues at Stanford and at Interleukin Genetics did get some interesting initial results.

Matching Genes to Diet

The lead investigator on the A TO Z collaboration with Inter-leukin was Gardner's Stanford colleague Dr. Mindy Dopler Nelson.[2] The researchers analyzed DNA from cheek swabs from 133 of the original 311 women who participated in the A TO Z Study. Women whose assigned diet matched their genotype lost 5.3 percent of their body weight at the end of a year as opposed to 2.3 percent for those whose genotype didn't match their diet. This result was highly statistically significant. Within the Atkins group, for example, those whose genotype matched the diet lost about 12 pounds compared to people without the low-carb genotype, who lost about two pounds. Results for the Ornish ultra-low-fat group were similar.

Low-carb vs. low-fat genotypes, by the way, run about 50-50.

Despite the fact that women whose genotype matched their diet lost almost five times as much weight as those who didn't, Gardner insists quite rightly that larger studies are needed.

My Personal Genotyping Experiment

If you go to the Internet you'll see that genotyping for weight—and for a lot of other stuff, including fitness, disease susceptibility, and cultural heritage—is already big business. You can even track the pattern of migration that your ancestors followed and locate distant relatives.

The ethical considerations that come up around genotyping are legion. If you have a gene that predisposes to disease, for example, could that affect your employability? What might happen if you, like Angelina Jolie, discover that you have a genetic propensity for breast cancer? Do you want to know or not?

Some genetic testing companies analyze your DNA and send you a report directly. Others require a physician as the intermediary. Because it can be difficult for a layperson to vet the results of genotyping, there's always the possibility of overreaction to an unexpected finding. Alternatively, some people might minimize a result that needs follow-up. For these reasons I suggest that if you plan to have genetic testing done, consider working with a company that sets up testing through a physician.

Food sleuth that I am, I decided to do just that.

My friend and colleague Sara Gottfried, M.D. (her book *The Hormone Cure* is excellent, by the way), had already been genotyped by Pathway Genomics out of San Diego. She had chosen their Pathway Fit diet, nutrition, and exercise personal genetic report and was able to order the same test for me. Here's an important informational bite. I have no professional relationship with Pathway Genomics. Whether you decide to get your testing done there or not makes no difference to me, financial or otherwise.

Using research provided by scientists from leading institutions like UC Berkeley, Harvard Medical School, Scripps Clinic, and others, Pathway Genomics tests about 75 genetic markers "to provide you with the latest, most comprehensive, and scientifically-advanced recommendations on diet, nutrition, exercise, addictive behaviors and weight-related health conditions."[3]

The goals of the Pathway Fit profile include optimizing metabolism, weight, exercise, and the nutritional balance of your diet. I was psyched. The DNA collection kit arrived at my door in good order. It was sturdy and aesthetically pleasing, and came with informed consent forms to fill out, notice of genetic counseling that the company provides for free, and specific directions on how to get a good harvest of epithelial cells (the source of the DNA that will be tested) in your saliva. Ten minutes of spitting later, the enclosed test tube was capped, packed, and ready for its journey back to the lab in San Diego.

Several weeks later the results of the test were sent both to me and to Dr. Sara. They came in a nice little booklet that outlined my genetic variations, what studies indicate their importance, and what I should do to optimize weight and wellness.

Should I eat a low-carb diet, a low-fat diet, a balanced diet of all three macronutrients, or a Mediterranean diet? Should I eat more unsaturated fats or monounsaturated fats like olive oil? What about saturated fats? Are they likely to raise my cholesterol or not? Am I predisposed to regain weight after dieting? If there's something yummy around, am I more or less likely to binge on it than other people? What exercise is best for me? And does exercise result in weight loss or not for my metabolic type? Am I predisposed to snacking? Am I normally or abnormally hungry? Do I have a sweet tooth? And—here's one I particularly enjoyed—how fast do I metabolize caffeine?

The test covers all those bases and many more.

Pathway Genomics tells you which studies have identified the genetic markers they test for, and also how robust the studies are. They rate them from one star (extremely preliminary) to four stars (large studies with at least 2,000 subjects that have been replicated at least once). Okay. That's cool.

I couldn't wait to see what type of diet they recommended for my metabolic type. I turned to page 8, filled with wide-eyed expectation. No doubt it would be the low-carb diet, since cutting back on carbs had pretty well cured everything that ailed me.

I turned the page, holding my breath. The suspense was soon over.

It said "Low Fat Diet: Your genotype is associated with weight loss or other health benefits from a diet lower in fats, especially saturated fats." According to the research they cited, I have a higher than average genetic risk for elevated LDL or "bad cholesterol," so they advised limiting saturated fat intake.

They cited seven studies to support their recommendation: one four-star study and six three-star studies. Pretty good. But once again there's a big slip between the cup and the lip. My LDL level has always been super low, a point of pride for my family practice doc. "Whatever you're doing, just keep on doing it" is her usual advice. Not only is my LDL not high. It's very low—the cardiologist's dream. I could live on a diet of butter (not really, but you get the drift) and my LDL level wouldn't budge.

So I was disappointed in the diet recommendation. But after my next blood test, I began to wonder if my specific genetic profile really did mean that I should eat less saturated fat. On a near Paleo diet, I had an LDL level that had indeed remained very low. But you may recall that LDL-C—total serum cholesterol—predicts heart disease only 50 percent of the time. Not very impressive. A better predictor is LDL-P, total number of cholesterol particles. The more particles you have in your blood, the more chance they'll bump up against the endothelium of your blood vessels, and if they're oxidized, start the process of clogging your arteries with plaque. My LDL-P was—gasp—borderline high. I was shocked.

Since most doctors still do not order tests to measure LDL-P, unfortunately, I had no baseline for comparison. When I was on the vegan diet, they hadn't been measured. My husband, Gordon, also turned out to have elevated LDL-P, which made his cardiologist extremely unhappy. "Meat is a condiment," she kept reminding him. Eat lots of vegetables, fruits, nuts, and good fats instead. So we both tweaked our diets to cut way back on meat and saturated fat.

Although the research tells us that good fats are healthful for the average person, it appears that neither of us is average. Our next set of blood tests will reveal whether cutting back on meat, eating more fish, going from full-fat to nonfat yogurt, moderating intake of hard cheese, and limiting butter to just a few pats a week reduces our LDL-P.

So, although the genetic testing was off base about the response of my LDL-C to diet, it might have been right in terms of LDL-P. At this point in time, however, there's no substitute for being your own diet sleuth and covering all the bases.

Personalizing Your Diet

Diet optimization through genetics is indeed a work in progress. Advances in lipid biochemistry, epigenetics (how environmental factors, including the food you eat, changes your gene expression), and the study of gut microbes are unfolding at warp speed.

As sexy as genetic testing might seem, your own lab tests and simple physical indicators (like weight, blood pressure, and your lipid profile) may be a more reliable way to personalize your diet for the time being. Gene activity is regulated by millions of different modifiers, many of which remain to be discovered. Furthermore, food itself moderates gene activity.

I am, however, very impressed by the part of the Pathway Fit profile that reports on micronutrients, predominantly vitamins. I've avoided taking vitamins and supplements for the most part, hoping to get them from a whole-foods, plant-based diet. But with genetic testing, a new science of personalized supplementation is on the horizon. For instance, I have a genetic variant (the T/T genotype) of a gene called MTHFR. Use your imagination to figure out what some researchers call it when they're not referring to it by its proper name: methylenetetrahydrofolate reductase.

This MTHFR variant is linked to low levels of vitamin B_2, or riboflavin. Low riboflavin levels are in turn associated with increased levels of *homocysteine*, a risk factor for heart disease and stroke. My homocysteine level (a lab test that I highly recommend) is in the middle of the range, but it could be lower. Pathway Fit suggests that I "optimize intake" of foods rich in riboflavin like milk, cheese, green leafy veggies, legumes, and lean meats. Since one study found that vitamin B_2 lowers homocysteine levels in T/T folks like me, I'm *considering* using it as a supplement.

The Pathway Fit profile also suggests that I might be deficient in vitamin B_{12}. When I was on a low-fat vegan diet, I did supplement with B_{12}, since it's found only in animal products like meat, fish, poultry, milk, and eggs. Since I have an A/G genotype of the FUT2-rs602662 gene (now that's a mouthful), without knowing from my doc that my vitamin B_{12} levels are actually high, I might have gone on B_{12} supplementation. For now, eating lots of leafy greens and other veggies has my methylation system purring like a well-tuned engine or a contented cat.

Folate and foliage come from the same root. Gotta eat those greens and lots of them. I was never much of a salad person, having grown up in the days when a salad consisted of a sorry-looking bowl of wilted iceberg lettuce with a slice of anemic tomato and a few dried-up rounds of cucumber on top. Those days are gone, at least in our house. You'll love the salads I'll teach you to make in Part IV. I can't believe how I actually *yearn* for them now that my metabolism isn't upset with an unreasonable amount of carbs.

I won't bore you with the rest of my genetic testing, other than to brag about the irrelevant fact that I possess a gene shared by most elite athletes, making me a potentially strong sprinter. That factoid is indeed irrelevant because I blew out my right knee sprinting years ago. Perhaps I lack a gene for moderation (that's a joke, folks), but the way things are going in the field of genetics and behavior, it might actually be true.

Genes and Eating Behavior

Dr. Sara and I had an interesting conversation with Michael P. Nova, M.D., chief medical officer of Pathway Genomics. He told us that the company surveyed 35,000 peer-reviewed papers to choose the genes they test for. About 1,000 papers a month are published in the field of genetic testing, and many of them are pertinent to diet and eating behavior, so the field is evolving at a very rapid pace indeed.

The diet recommendations in the Pathway Fit test, we were told, were based on algorithms drawn from seven sectors. They don't believe in basing recommendations for type of diet on one gene and its variants. Fifty-five genes are actually surveyed to match you to one of their four diet types.

Pathway Genomics is especially impressive because of its concern for behavioral factors. It's one thing to know what type of diet might best suit your metabolic type. It's another thing entirely to have the discipline to implement dietary changes over the long haul.

Their first customer, in fact, was *The Biggest Loser* show. Pathway Genomics genotyped 300 extremely overweight people for them and found some highly specific behavioral markers. For example, you may have a taste receptor that makes broccoli repellent. Or you may have a sweet tooth. Or like me, you may have trouble moderating your intake if a very tasty food is around, a trait they refer to as "eating disinhibition."

No package of potato chips is safe around me, which is why we don't keep them in the house.

When I asked Dr. Nova whether genotyping could help predict who might develop metabolic syndrome, he told us that the company was currently developing an algorithm for that. They're also developing testing around sugar metabolism to indicate people at higher risk for developing diabetes. As time goes on and new research pours in, genetic testing is likely to become more and more valuable and to include the microbiome (the genetic code of our gut microbes), which the Nestle company reputedly put a billion dollars into sequencing.

It makes sense that weight and genetics are related. But the really big surprise in weight control and metabolism is . . . c'mon, I know you've been waiting for this . . . the 100 trillion friendly microbes that make your gut their home. Stay tuned for the latest on the microbiome (your gut bacteria and their genes) in the next chapter.

CHAPTER 14

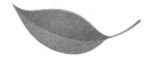

Gut Microbes:

The Metabolic Surprise
of the Millennium

*"The Hygiene Hypothesis—or Old Friends Hypothesis,
if you prefer—posits that a great many diseases
(specifically autoimmune diseases) result from a disconnect
with the natural world and its myriad of microscopic life."*

— JEFF LEACH, MICROBIOLOGIST AND FOUNDER
OF THE HUMAN FOOD PROJECT

Back in 2006 Jeffrey Gordon, M.D., and his colleagues at the Washington University School of Medicine in St. Louis published a paper in the journal *Nature* demonstrating that thin mice and obese mice have different populations of gut bacteria. Furthermore, they proved that one particular type of bacteria caused obesity, rather than obesity changing the types of bacteria. When the scientists isolated a strain of Firmicutes bacteria from chubby mice, and then introduced them into the bacteria-free guts of thin mice raised in a sterile environment, the skinny mice fattened up in just 10 to 14 days.[1]

Mice aren't the only species that harbor thrifty Firmicutes bacteria. Humans do, too. And just like mice, those of us who co-exist with Firmicutes as part of our gut ecosystem are more likely to be fat. One of my Facebook followers was thrilled to hear this news. She posted a tearful response, writing that she hoped to live long enough to tell all the people who torment her about her weight—even though she's a healthy eater—that it really isn't her fault.

I felt a lot of compassion for her. How frustrating it must be to eat very little and look like you're sneaking donuts in the night. If that's your problem and someone starts in about your weight, try this line: "Hey, it's not my fault. The Firmicutes did it." That should put a graceful end to the conversation. But perhaps we don't know enough about the complex causes of obesity to blame it all on the Firmicutes, although they may be part of the overall picture.

What If Overeating Is a Symptom, but Not the Cause, of Obesity?

When I told a friend about some of the research on gut bacteria and obesity, she was duly skeptical. "I have some obese friends, and bacteria or no, they just plain eat too much," she offered.

"While that could be true," I countered (thinking about the Fat-Storage Trifecta that you learned about in Chapter 9), "overeating may not be the fundamental reason *why* they're overweight. The more weight a person carries, the less leptin (the satiety hormone) they secrete and the hungrier they'll be. It's like their off-switch is broken. So what if overeating is a symptom, but not the main *cause*, of obesity that's caused by something else? I'm not saying this is true in *every* case because obesity is a complicated condition. But I do think that gut bacteria may revolutionize the way we think about weight. The question is: Can we change the composition of our community of gut bacteria, and will people lose weight when that happens?"

Naturally, researchers and Big Pharma are hot to answer that question.

Thrifty Firmicutes

Those clever Firmicutes that Dr. Gordon and his colleagues studied are experts in extracting calories from food. They're good friends to have around in times of famine when you might have to fill your belly with some pretty fibrous stuff like leaves, stems, or even bark. The Firmicutes possess a rare metabolic talent that allows them to digest the complex sugars that fibrous vegetation contains, breaking them down into small, digestible components.

Dr. Gordon's colleague Vanessa Ridaura carried out a landmark study of gut bacteria present in identical pairs of human female twins where one was thin and the other was fat. Twin studies are popular because the genetic influence on metabolism is controlled for. These were her findings:

> When gut bacteria from a lean human twin were transferred into mice raised in sterile environments, the mice stayed thin. But when thin mice raised in a sterile environment received bacterial transplants from an obese twin, they got fat.[2]

It took the latter rodents a mere five weeks to gain 15 to 17 percent more weight than their peers.

One of the star researchers in the field of nutrition and gut microbes is Dr. Patrice Cani, a professor at Catholic University in Louvain, Belgium. His lab tracks the interaction between gut bacteria, metabolism, and obesity. His research has revealed that when obese mice (that have been fed a high-fat diet) are fed a prebiotic (a fiber nutrient that certain strains of bacteria like to eat), the number of a species of mucin-degrading bacteria called *A. muciniphila* increases markedly. As a result, the rodents lose almost half their body fat without any change to their diet. Their insulin resistance also disappears.[3]

Fat, Fiber, and Leaky Gut

> Hippocrates, the father of modern medicine, once said that all disease begins in the gut. Amazing as that may seem, he may well be correct.

When mice are fed a high-fat diet to make them obese, they promptly develop a syndrome called *leaky gut*. Normally the junctions between the cells that line your digestive tract are tight to prevent bacterial toxins and bits of unprocessed food or poop from getting into your body. (Yuck!)

If the tight junctions loosen up—the equivalent of a circle of people who are holding hands letting go—then bits of bacteria, food, poop, or other stuff that is normally kept inside the gut can sneak into your circulation. When bits of bacterial cell membrane leak through the gut lining, the immune system mounts an attack that can also target one's own cells—a condition known as *auto-immune disease.*

Inflammation, insulin resistance, metabolic syndrome, and type 2 diabetes may also be—at least in part—the result of leaky gut.

The gut harbors several varieties of gram-negative bacteria, some of which are good guys and some of which are bad guys. The cell membranes of all gram-negative bacteria are composed in part of structural molecules called lipopolysaccharides (LPS), consisting of a lipid molecule joined to a polysaccharide (sugar).

LPS molecules are *endotoxins*, molecules that stimulate a powerful immune response if they penetrate the gut wall and get into the circulation.[4] Not only can they cause autoimmune disease and potentially fatal *endotoxemia* (poisoning by the endotoxins), but as we'll discuss shortly, they may also be the elephant in the room of depression.

Dietary Fat and Leaky Gut

Okay. So if rats fed a high-fat diet develop leaky gut, obesity, inflammation, and metabolic problems, what does that mean for us humans? Is fat the bad guy after all? Are my Paleo friends, some of whom eat quite a lot of fat, doomed to metabolic meltdown? And since Gordie and I were eating a substantial amount of saturated fat before our LDL-P levels led us to cut back, could our own guts have developed leaks midsteak?

Jeff Leach, bacterial anthropologist and founder of the Human Food Project (www.humanfoodproject.com), wrote an illuminating blog post about bacteria and leaky gut entitled "Can a High-Fat Paleo Diet Cause Obesity and Diabetes?"

Reflecting on studies in which mice were fed a high-fat diet that caused weight gain, inflammation, insulin resistance, and ultimately type 2 diabetes, Leach focused on the protective effects of friendly microbes known as Bifidobacterium.

The fiber oligofructose from chicory root is known to stimulate the growth of Bifidobacterium. Leach reviews the results of a study that looked at the interaction between fat and fiber:

> The fiber was added to a high-fat diet fed to one group of mice, but not to the same high-fat diet fed to another group. In the high-fat-only group, endotoxemia was significantly increased, but in the high-fat diet that also included the prebiotic, Bifidobacterium levels predictably went up and the LPS levels were normalized. This also correlated with improved glucose tolerance and a normalized inflammatory "tone."[5]

> Bifidobacterium are metabolic heroes. They synthesize the short-chain fatty acids butyrate, propionate, and lactate, which nourish the gut epithelium, protect the integrity of tight junctions, and keep the gut barrier intact. To perform their magic, Bifidobacteria need prebiotics (fiber that feeds them) from onion, garlic, dandelion greens, chicory root, and tubers like Jerusalem artichokes. Americans get only one to four grams of those prebiotics, on average, daily.

Leach continues:

> If in fact the levels of Bifidobacterium in our microbiota mediate gut permeability . . . then our chronic low intake of prebiotic dietary fibers may be a significant player in our epidemic of metabolic syndrome. It is interesting to think that all of the attention that has been given to various substances that might lead to a leaky gut might be missing the 800-pound gorilla in the room—Bifidobacterium. Think I will have onion and garlic with my dinner tonight—how about you?[6]

Yes, indeedy. We have onion for dinner on most nights, Jeff. While an apple a day may keep the doctor away, an apple and an onion a day—plus a really big plate full of greens—may be even better.

Leach makes the point that the government *MyPlate* dietary recommendation is way behind the times. We need to eat a *BioPlate* instead. That sage advice is based on the fact that the usual government dietary advice ignores the rather astounding fact that 90 percent of our cells aren't even human. They're bacterial. And they're hungry, too.

The number of good bacteria in the gut can be increased in a couple of ways. The host can eat foods or take supplements rich in the prebiotics that the bacteria prefer, or bacteria can be grown in a broth and then fed directly to the host.

Now there's an interesting fantasy. Drink a bowl of soup and get skinny. It would appear that we may not be as far as you might think from just such an amazing breakthrough. There is, however, yet another way to enrich our gut with beneficial microbes. They're called *fecal transplants*, which are exactly what they sound like. I hope you weren't eating when you read that.

Fecal Implants

A 2013 study out of the Netherlands, published in the prestigious *New England Journal of Medicine,* prepared fecal solutions from healthy volunteers and placed them in the small intestine of patients infected with *Clostridium difficile,* the notorious *C. diff* that kills about 13,000 Americans annually. *C. diff* can be exceptionally difficult to eradicate even with powerful antibiotics like vancomycin. The results of the fecal transplant were spectacular. The bacterial implant cured the infection in over 85 percent of recipients—a much higher rate than antibiotic therapy.[7] For those whose transplant didn't vanquish the *C. diff* infection the first time around, a second transplant usually did the trick.

An earlier 2012 study out of the same group in the Netherlands investigated the role that bacteria might play in reversing metabolic syndrome. They infused intestinal microbes from thin people (with normal metabolism) into male recipients with metabolic syndrome. *Take note. This isn't about mice. It's about us.* Then they studied the effect of the transplants on the composition of the recipients' microbiome and on their glucose metabolism. Six weeks after the infusion, the insulin sensitivity of the recipients had increased significantly. The researchers concluded that intestinal microbes might be developed as therapeutic agents to increase insulin sensitivity.[8]

Bacteria, Leaky Gut, and Depression

Anxiety, depression, autism spectrum disorders (ASD), attention deficit hyperactivity disorder (ADHD), schizophrenia, and a host of neurological, mental health, and mood disorders are related, at least in part, to our gut microbes. While reviewing the burgeoning literature on mind and microbes is beyond the scope of this book, I do want to mention one condition—depression—and relate it to the health of our children.

Feeding your kids low-fiber foods high in bad fats—oxidized fats, trans fats, polyunsaturated fats like supermarket-brand oils, processed-cheese spreads or slices, and commercial pizza made with cheap "analog cheese" whipped up by food chemists to mimic the characteristics of real mozzarella—increases the possibility that they will develop leaky gut syndrome. Once thought to be a fiction that circulated largely in the alternative medical community, even mainstream physicians now know that leaky gut is a real phenomenon linked to a host of immune-related, inflammatory conditions, including depression.

Checked out a school lunch lately? When the food we give our kids is fake food (what Michael Pollan calls *Foodlike Substances*), we're altering the environment of their gut bacteria, starving out some of the good guys, and setting up the conditions for both obesity and leaky gut, as well as planting the seeds of depression and anxiety.

The millennials (born between 1977 and 1992) are reported to be the most stressed, depressed, and anxious generation in recent history. Yes, they're under a lot of pressure, living in a world of unpredictable change, scarce jobs, and electronic communication. The latter can trump the all-important face-to-face connectivity that stabilizes our brain and immune system. But the younger generations are also victims of the fake-food legacy.

According to journalist Ann Brown, "Depression has been diagnosed for 19 percent of millennials, compared with 14 percent of Generation X (ages 34 to 47); 12 percent of Baby Boomers (ages 48 to 66); and 11 percent of those ages 67 and older. Anxiety disorder has also been cited in millennials more than other generations, 12 percent, compared with 8 percent of Gen X, 7 percent of Boomers, and 4 percent of seniors."[9]

> It's humbling to think that depression and anxiety are related to our gut bacteria perhaps as much as to our mothers, Freud notwithstanding. But one thing you can bet on is that as moms become more nutritionally literate, their kids will get healthier both in mind and body. One of the ways moms might accomplish that is by caring for their children's microbes with the same reverent attention given to their soccer practices and volleyball matches.

"Not to sound cavalier," Leach writes, "but nutrition and disease is this generation's civil rights movement; let's start treating it accordingly."[10]

A New Look at Fiber

Pretty soon, if Leach is right, our young folks will be holding up placards demanding more fiber in their diet. Back in the old days of nutritional literacy, we all knew that eating lots of fiber makes for plumper, more regular poops. But a new look at fiber shows that it does a whole lot more than gear up your guts.

All plant foods contain fiber, which Jeff Leach defines as "any part of a plant that cannot be digested and absorbed in the small intestine and ends up in the large bowel (colon). Once in the colon, dietary fiber is broken down and utilized by our good bugs for their own growth and turned into energy (calories) for us."[11]

> Like people with individual metabolic needs, various strains of bacteria also thrive on different types of fiber. That's why a diversity of vegetables, fruits, beans, and whole grains (for those of us who can eat the latter two foods) cultivate healthy bacterial growth.

Unfortunately, the microbiome of most modern Americans is a rather pitiful shadow of what it might be. The average adult American eats only 12 to 15 grams of fiber a day. According to an Institute of Medicine formula based on getting 14 grams of fiber for every 1,000 calories, women are supposed to eat 25 grams per day and men 38 grams. According to ethnographic and fossil data, combined with studies of contemporary hunter-gather populations, the government recommendations are off by several orders of magnitude. *Aiming for 100 grams of fiber or more daily would be a lot more beneficial.*

Oligofructose and inulin are types of fiber found in garlic, onions, yams, chicory root, bananas, wheat, the tuber known as a Jerusalem artichoke, dandelion greens, leeks, and jicama. You can't get away with taking a fiber pill that contains just a single source of fiber, though. Only by eating a variety of whole-plant foods can you increase the biodiversity of your gut bacterial community.

Some people have asked me about the GAPS diet (Gut and Psychology Syndrome) for leaky gut and autoimmune disease. It limits the intake of certain kinds of fiber. As far as I know, this diet hasn't been researched. But because it's a whole-foods, plant-based diet, it's likely to be beneficial—but perhaps for reasons other than specifying particular types of fiber. Any whole-foods diet is better than a processed-food diet. You, of course, are the experimenter-in-chief of your own domain. If you want to experiment with different types of fiber, by all means knock yourself out. The experiment will certainly make you more mindful, as well as more regular.

This is the bottom line: The less processed any food is, and the more fiber it contains, the better it is for your gut microbes and therefore for you. Furthermore, the kind of food you eat is a powerful modifier not only of your microbial community and its genes (your microbiome) but also of the community of your mammalian cells and their genes. More about that in the next chapter.

CHAPTER 15

Epigenetics:

How the Environment Controls Our Genes

"Genes load the gun, and environment pulls the trigger."

— Francis Collins, M.D., PhD.,
director of the National Institutes of Health

The past ten years have been a time of great change in science. In the last Science Bite, you read about the microbial revolution. In this Bite, we'll turn our attention to the genetic revolution. In 1958 Francis Crick, who discovered the structure of DNA along with Dr. James Watson, formulated what was referred to as the Central Dogma of Molecular Biology: DNA makes RNA makes protein.

Genes are made of DNA, and their job is to code for the production of proteins (through the intermediary of RNA) that the body needs as building blocks, enzymes, and other molecules necessary for life.

Genes were once synonymous with potential. If you had good genes, that was terrific. If you had bad genes, watch out. But the worm has turned. Dr. Francis Collins, who was leader of the Human Genome Project before he became director of the National Institutes of Health (NIH), was referring to the new field of epigenetics (a word that means "above the genes") when he stated that genes load the gun, but the environment pulls the trigger.

> The foods that we eat are powerful epigenetic regulators, triggers that determine whether our genes express their potential for either health or disease.

A TALE (TAIL?) OF TWO MICE: PART ONE

Dr. Dana Dolinoy, at the University of Michigan School of Public Health, did an interesting experiment demonstrating how food and chemicals can change gene expression. Check out her short talk "Epigenetics; or Why DNA Is Not Your Destiny" (www.youtube.com/watch?v=D9CzvalZ2zY).

In ten minutes, Dr. Dolinoy explains what the field of epigenetics is all about and introduces her audience (hopefully you) to the *Tale of Two Sisters*, identical twins from the same mouse mother. One sister is obese, has a yellow coat, and is diabetic. Her sister is lean, has a brown coat, and has normal metabolism. What makes the difference? Stay tuned for a few basics, and then I'll let you in on the secret to this intriguing mystery in Part Two of a *Tale of Two Sisters*.

Down and Dirty with the Epigenome

> Let's start by further defining epigenetics. The human genome is fairly constant and changes very slowly over millions of years. On the other hand, the environment around us changes all the time. The new science of epigenetics explains how our genes can adapt to changes in the environment even though the actual structure of the genome—the genes themselves—don't change.

What *does* change is whether or not certain genes are accessible to the gene-reading machinery within the cell. Think of human DNA as very long strands. Every tiny cell in your body houses 1.8 meters of DNA, which is almost 6 feet! All that DNA would be a tangled mess were it not for a biological spool of four *histone* proteins that form an octomer around which the DNA wraps itself. The histone spool and its associated DNA is called a *nucleosome*. The histone molecules have tails that flop over the coiled strand of DNA and either tighten the coils or loosen them.

Tightly coiled DNA is inaccessible for transcription (that is where RNA comes in), which means that the genes in that coil become silenced. Methyl molecules (CH_3) attach to the histones and tighten the coils of DNA, blocking access to genes. Acetyl molecules ($COCH_3$), on the other hand, loosen the coils of DNA, making genes available and open for business. The methyl and acetyl groups are called epigenetic *marks*. These marks—and several others that are beyond the scope of this discussion—act as switches that turn genes on and off in response to environmental changes.

DNA itself can also be methylated to silence genes that aren't needed in different types of cells. That's what allows specialization in structure and function. While all our cells have the same DNA, it's not all active; otherwise, there would be no difference between a hair cell, an ovum, a neuron, or a fat cell. The DNA in all our genes is identical. The difference comes about through which genes are active and which are turned off.

The sum total of epigenetic marks controls your gene activity. As I already mentioned, epigenetics technically means "above the genes," and that's just what the marks represent—a control panel. That panel is called the *epigenome.*

Proper methylation is indispensable for healthy metabolism, which means that the body has to produce a ready supply of molecular intermediaries to maintain the methylation apparatus. Those come from the foods that we eat. For an excellent review of the subject, read the discussion by functional physician Mark Hyman, M.D., at http://drhyman.com/blog/2011/02/08 /maximizing-methylation-the-key-to-healthy-aging-2/#close.

Methylation repairs DNA, is indispensable to the detoxification process in the body, and is required for healthy aging. Diabetes and Alzheimer's disease, for instance, are both associated with deranged patterns of methylation. Enzymes called methyl transferases are critical to how the process works. SAM, sometimes written as SAMe (S-adenosylmethionine), is a dietary compound sold in health-food stores as a mood stabilizer. It works with an enzyme called DNA-methyltransferase to donate methyl groups to DNA.

SAM also occurs naturally in your body. When you eat sesame seeds, Brazil nuts, fish, peppers, or spinach, those foods contribute methionine to SAM biosynthesis. Folic acid or folate (you may recall that *folate* comes from the same root as *foliage*) occurs in leafy green vegetables and also feeds into the methylation system. Vitamin B_{12} in egg yolks, meat, shellfish, and liver, and vitamin B_6 in meats, vegetables, and nuts also contribute to the synthesis of methionine, which feeds into the SAM cycle, assuring methylation.

If you're a vegan, problems with methylation can lead to big trouble. Since vitamin B_{12} is indispensable to the methylation process—and comes from eating egg yolks, fish, liver, and meat—long-term veganism can result in serious health problems unless you very carefully supplement your diet with vitamin B_{12}.

You Are a Petri Dish Covered with Skin

When I was a cell biologist, I grew cancer cells in petri dishes. They grow in a nutrient mixture called growth medium, in an incubator heated to body temperature. I was experimenting with changes in the growth medium to investigate whether a different nutrient mix would alter the *phenotype* of the cells.

The phenotype is how a cell looks and acts. The short story is that I could change cellular appearance and behavior by changing the kind of fatty acids added to the growth medium. The genetic makeup of the cells (the *genotype*) stayed the same, but the components of the growth medium made the difference between the cells looking and acting normal or looking and acting like cancer cells.

Our human bodies are like petri dishes covered with skin. The medium that nourishes our cells is constantly changing in response to the environment.

For example, if you feel stressed, your body releases a host of hormones and neurotransmitters, including adrenaline, pro-inflammatory cytokines, and cortisol—which, by the way, causes the accumulation of belly fat.

If you're loved and cared for, your body produces hormones like oxytocin, which promotes bonding, and endorphins that create pleasure and relieve pain. When you see something beautiful, or when news of a disaster saddens you, once again your growth medium reflects your changing emotional responses.

Epigenetic Inheritance

My friend and colleague, cell biologist Bruce Lipton, Ph.D., wrote a best-selling book entitled *The Biology of Belief.* Indeed, what we believe and how those beliefs shape our emotions, behavior, and experience of life makes a world of difference to our health through the elegance of epigenetic pathways.

But here's the big news. Not only do epigenetic changes affect us, but they also affect our children, and in some instances our grandchildren and great-grandchildren.

If a pregnant woman is stressed, the changes in her growth medium also affect the cells of her developing child. For example, babies born to moms who were traumatized by the destruction of the World Trade Center on 9/11 are more likely to have an exaggerated response to stressful situations, including strangers, new foods, or loud noises.

A pregnant mom's nutrition is also important to the baby's development.

Prenatal diets low in folate, or folic acid; vitamin B_{12}; and other foods containing methyl groups can lead to a variety of health issues for the baby. These include cleft palate, brain and spinal cord defects, asthma, and behavioral problems.

Moms who eat a lot of junk food when they're pregnant or nursing are setting up their children for a lifetime of addiction to such foods.[1,2] Research done in Australia with rats demonstrated that junk foods high in sugar and fat increase the release of opioids and the reward-seeking hormone dopamine in the brain. The dopamine circuit creates the cravings that keep you going back for more. When rat dams were fed sugary cereal, meat patties, potato chips, and peanut butter, their diet altered the pups' gene expression so that the little rats were more likely to prefer eating junk food as they matured.

Dr. Mühlhäusler, one of the researchers, commented, "The take-home message for women is that eating large amounts of junk food during pregnancy and while breastfeeding will have long-term consequences for their child's preference for these foods, which will ultimately have negative effects on their health."[3]

A fascinating aspect of epigenetics is that while most of the marks are erased during gametogenesis—when eggs and sperm differentiate—a small percentage of the marks remain active and are therefore inherited by the offspring, and potentially by their offspring, for several generations.

I'm Jewish, and three out of my four grandparents immigrated to the United States from Eastern Europe where their families endured the terror of pogroms for many generations. Twelve of my family members were killed in Auschwitz, and I grew up in fear of a similar fate. I always wondered why I have an exaggerated response to stress. Epigenetics helped me understand that. The fear circuits in my brain were literally shaped by the stress that my ancestors endured. *This particular kind of epigenetic effect—that of stress—can be handed down for three or four generations.*

Famine also creates heritable epigenetic marks. Food was scarce in Holland near the end of World War II. In the winter of 1944, the Germans worsened the situation when they imposed a food embargo, and 30,000 people starved to death. Pregnant women who survived the famine had very small babies. While that stands to reason, when those babies grew up and had children of their own, their babies were also small even though the moms were well nourished. The offspring also suffered from a range of disorders, including diabetes, obesity, coronary artery disease, and breast and other cancers. Some of these changes persisted in the grandchildren of the original famine survivors.

But trauma and starvation aren't the only kind of stress that can leave epigenetic marks on the genome. Environmental toxins can do the same. University of Texas zoologist David Crews and his colleagues have done research showing that a single exposure to a fungicide (vinclozolin) in rats affects the stress response of their offspring three generations down the line.[4]

Many of the pesticides, herbicides, fungicides, and other chemicals used to grow crops are likely to have epigenetic effects. This is the reason why, if you can manage it financially, eating organic food is so important—especially any food containing fat (think dairy, eggs, meats, and oils), in which pesticide and chemical residues are concentrated.

A TALE (TAIL?) OF TWO MICE: PART TWO

This brings us back to the tale of Dr. Dolinoy's twin sister mice. One, as you may recall, was yellow, obese, and diabetic. The other was slim, brown, and had normal metabolism. These mice carry a gene called the agouti gene. If it's unmethylated, you get a yellow mouse whose agouti gene is always turned on. It's hungry, gets fat, and develops diabetes. The slim brown sister's agouti gene is methylated and therefore silenced. She doesn't overeat and maintains normal metabolism.

Now the plot thickens. The twin sister mice were born to a mother who was exposed to bisphenol A (BPA) during her pregnancy. BPA is a compound found in plastic baby bottles, water bottles, food containers, the linings of cans, bottle tops, and some dental sealants. BPA is an endocrine disrupter that mimics the effect of estrogen. It also disturbs methylation in the developing fetus. The result is that some of the baby mice from the same litter are born yellow, others are brown, and still others are hybrids with an agouti gene that is only partially silenced.

Now this is the big news, **so listen up**. If the mama's diet is supplemented with genistein, the major phytonutrient in soy, at levels equivalent to eating a diet high in soy protein for a human being, the agouti genes of her babies are more likely to be methylated, so more healthy brown mice get born.[5]

I'm not necessarily suggesting that you eat soy. I *am* suggesting that you eat a wide variety of vegetables and greens for their important epigenetic effects. It's also wise to watch out for plastics where food is concerned. At the very least, look for BPA-free plastic bags (Ziploc is one brand), and BPA-free cans, and use glass or stainless-steel food containers instead of plastic ones. Plastic still leaches endocrine disruptors other than BPA, but you've got to pick your battles.

Now you know enough about your microbiome and your epigenome to understand more clearly why one diet can't suit everyone. You're acquainted with the practicalities of eating a plant-based diet rich in fiber, greens, and vegetables that contribute to methylation. (Yes, I know that this is a lot of information and that it might help to reread these Science Bites a couple of times.)

In the next Bite, we'll get to the most practical way of personalizing your diet. While all of us will be healthier if we eat a high-fiber, plant-based diet, we vary considerably in how much carbohydrate our bodies can process without creating oxidative stress, inflammation, obesity, and metabolic disturbances. That's why instead of thinking in terms of high-carb or low-carb diets, I like to think in terms of eating a carb-reasonable diet. Read on and you'll discover what carb-reasonable means for you.

CHAPTER 16

Going Carb-Reasonable

"The more easily digestible and refined the carbohydrates, the greater the effect on our health, weight and well-being."

— ANDREW WEIL, M.D.

Life is not fair. I'll bet you know someone who munches upon bonbons, drinks Cokes, eats pizza, thrives on submarine sandwiches, and is rail thin and vibrantly healthy—refined carbs be damned. These people are especially frustrating to those of us who can gain weight just from walking past a bakery.

If you want to read a funny and informative blog about this subject, Peter Attia, M.D., has a cool one on his site, The Eating Academy. It's worth reading because he's such a good scientist (just obsessive enough to teach really well and funny enough to make it interesting), and a talented statistician who knows his numbers.

Dr. Attia is an elite athlete who, when he set out to lose some weight, was used to exercising for about four hours a day. Even with that, he was about 50 pounds overweight. No, let me repeat, life is *not* fair. His wife wondered if he could become a "little less not thin."

The good Dr. Attia was fit but still fat.

According to his fascinating account, he just has to look at carbs and he starts storing fat:

> On the other hand, my wife can eat a bag of Oreo cookies for dinner every night, coupled with all the pasta, bread, and rice the world has to offer and not put on one pound. . . . How is this possible? Does this mean insulin doesn't control fat metabolism? **No, it means we have an entirely different genetic make-up.** Her grandmother is 86 years old, eats bread all day long, is healthy as a horse, and weighs 100 pounds. Conversely, I come from a family where every single man has died of heart disease and looked like the Pillsbury Dough Boy prior to doing so.[1]

Dr. Attia's description of his family history suggests a genetic variation in metabolism that leads to insulin resistance and metabolic syndrome unless carbs are seriously restricted. There are no if, ands, or buts about it. When he ate an athlete's high-carb diet, he got fat. He was carrying around 50 extra pounds in spite of eating what he thought was a healthy diet and exercising like a demon for several hours each day. You can see the before-and-after pictures and read his interesting and entertaining story at http://eatingacademy.com/my-personal-nutrition-journey.

A Hypothetical Carb-Tolerance Spectrum

In one of his other blog posts, Dr. Attia estimates that 10 to 20 percent of the population are similar to his thin wife.[2] They "maintain exquisite insulin sensitivity" even when they eat carloads of carbs. On the other hand, he suggests that 30 to 40 percent of the population is exquisitely carb sensitive. In order to lose weight and normalize their metabolic markers, this group has to squeeze almost all the carbs out of their diet. The rest of us are somewhere in the middle of the carb-sensitivity spectrum.

> The average American eats a humongous 350 grams of carbs a day, most of them low-GI, fiber-poor carbs that result in surges of glucose, insulin resistance, and increased fat storage. Your 100 trillion microbial buddies don't enjoy that diet, either. *In contrast, both the United States Department of Agriculture and the Institute of Medicine recommend 130 grams of carbs per day for both adults and children.*

I'm one of the middling carb-sensitivity folks. Just for fun imagine a bell curve with the suggested average of 130 grams of carbs as the top of the bell, smack in the middle of the curve.[3]

To reboot metabolism, as we've already discussed, the most carb-resistant folks will do best in terms of both weight loss and metabolic markers by sticking initially to the far left side of the curve, eating fewer than 50 grams of carbs per day. People like Dr. Attia's wife—and perhaps those who still resemble string beans long after adolescence has passed—can eat more than 130 grams of carbs and reside at the far right of the curve.

Yes, I know that the curve is not really symmetrical with an equal number of people falling either to the right of center (carb tolerant) or to the left (carb resistant), but for the sake of expedience, we'll think of it that way so that you can get an idea of what eating a low-, medium-, or high-carb-reasonable PlantPlus Diet might look like.

Glycemic Load and Glycemic Index

I typically eat somewhere between 50 and 75 obvious grams of carbs a day. That might not sound like many, but like David Perlmutter, M.D., and Chris Kresser, I don't bother to count the carbs in low-starch vegetables like cauliflower and broccoli, greens, carrots, celery, onions, summer squash, green beans, cabbage, fennel, and the like. Those carbs are burned slowly, feeding your microbiome rather than your fat pads.

When people ask whether I'm on a low-carb diet, my answer is not at all. I like to think in terms of a carb-reasonable, low-glycemic-load diet instead. Glycemic index (GI) measures how fast foods break down into sugar in your blood. The higher the GI, the more quickly the food spikes sugar and insulin—turning on the fat-storage machinery. Starchy foods like white potatoes are a case in point. They're nearly equivalent to eating table sugar.

What the GI doesn't tell you is *how much* carb you're getting in an actual *serving* of food. This is important since we eat food portions rather than charts. The GI of watermelon, for example, is very high. But its Glycemic Load (GL) per portion is extremely low because watermelon is mostly water by weight. It doesn't have many carbs in each serving.

Wikipedia has a concise definition of glycemic load:

> The **glycemic load (GL)** of food is a number that estimates how much the food will raise a person's blood glucose level after eating it. One unit of glycemic load approximates the effect of consuming one gram of glucose. Glycemic load accounts for how much carbohydrate is in the food and how much each gram of carbohydrate in the food raises blood glucose levels. Glycemic load is based on the glycemic index (GI), and is defined as the fraction of available carbohydrate in the food times the food's GI.

Unless you really love numbers, you won't be hanging out in front of the fridge making this calculation. Fortunately, there are lots of charts that do that for you. I like to study charts—just a couple of peeks helps a lot—to get a "feel" for where foods fall on the GL. You can Google various "Charts on Glycemic Load." Harvard Medical School put out a simple one featuring 100 common foods at: www.health.harvard.edu/newsweek/Glycemic_index_and_glycemic_load_for_100_foods.htm.

A few highlights follow.

Whoa—How Many Carbs Are in That?

Here's a fun fact. You already know that fruit juice spikes blood sugar, but when you eyeball the fact that the GL of apple juice is almost twice the GL of a Coke, that gets you thinking. Here are a few GLs of common foods for comparison that I pulled from the Harvard chart. The foods least likely to spike your blood sugar have a GL of 10 or less. But just because GL is low, that doesn't mean that the food in question is necessarily good for you:

- Frozen white bagel = 25 **versus** Aunt Jemima Frozen Waffles = 10

- Apple juice = 30 **versus** Coke = 16

- Instant oatmeal = 30 **versus** whole cooked oatmeal = 13

- White rice = 43 **versus** couscous = 9

- Reduced-fat yogurt with fruit = 13 **versus** premium ice cream = 3

- Banana = 16 **versus** apple = 6

- White spaghetti = 26 **versus** chickpeas = 3

- Fruit rollups = 24 **versus** Peanut M&M's = 6

Really? Ice cream and Peanut M&M's are low-GL foods? Yes, because the fat in the cream and in the peanuts slows absorption of the carbs. You can't use GL alone to guide healthful food choices, but if you're planning to eat junk food, you can at least minimize the blood-sugar spikes.

Remember, the more glucose on the loose (the higher the GL), the more insulin the average person releases and the more fat gets stored. But although you know that all calories are not created equal, if you stray from eating whole foods, the calories in processed foods count. Otherwise there'd surely be an ice cream, Peanut M&M, Coca-Cola diet plan.

Fiber-rich low-GL carbs are essential for the health of your gut microbes. As you may recall, microbes in your colon (particularly the Bifidobacterium and Lactobacillus that yogurt has made famous) need resistant fiber to ferment into short-chain fatty acids like acetate, butyrate, and propionate, which nourish the epithelial lining of the colon and prevent leaky gut, which can lead to inflammatory bowel disease, general inflammation, and autoimmune disease.

These good prebiotic carbs, by the way, don't show up in traditional carb counts since the *net carbs* in any food are calculated by deducting grams of fiber from total carbohydrate content. A medium apple, for example, has about 14 grams of net carbs once you deduct the 4 grams of fiber.

Once again, peeping at a carb chart a few times (Atkins makes a nice little booklet) can help you understand what you're eating. In just a few days of checking the foods you choose for carbs or GL, you'll start to understand where the carbs are. Then you can forget about counting and just focus on whole foods that have lots of fiber.

Why Is Carb Resistance So Variable?

Is there some easy indicator of how many carbs fit your metabolic type? What about blood type or country of origin?

When I first announced to friends, both real and virtual, that I was writing a book on personalized nutrition, several of them mentioned the blood-type diet, popularized by nutritionist Peter D'Adamo. While he has a fascinating hypothesis—that your blood type reflects the ancestral environment in which your forebears developed and that certain foods are thereby preferable for different blood types—the facts are more complex.

I really like his hypothesis, which predates most of the books out there on the importance of eating ancestral-type diets. It makes intuitive sense that populations who lived in specific environments—all of whom may initially have had the same blood type—had to adapt to burning the macronutrients that were most readily available.

You wouldn't expect an Eskimo to thrive on a relatively carb-rich diet of tubers, honey, fruits, leafy greens, nuts, and bush meat like hunter-gatherers in Africa do. The metabolic furnace of Eskimos developed under the influence of a frigid environment with a very limited growing season. They thrive on meat, fish, and oil-rich blubber.

If you're an Inuit who was raised in a traditional village in the Yukon and recently moved to Nome or Fairbanks, ancestral genetics are still vitally important. If an Inuit moves to the city and starts to eat pizza, pasta, potato chips, candy bars, soda, and the Standard American junk-food diet, they're likely to get sick pretty quickly. Within months such individuals gain significant weight, as well as become prediabetic and insulin resistant. If they go back to eating their ancestral foods, however, their health is restored.

But most of us are mongrels whose ancestors interbred over time and migrated in complex patterns over the face of the earth. No matter what our blood type is, our ancestral gene pool is more of a crap shoot. So discovering what we burn best is usually a process of careful observation and testing. My grandparents or at least their grandparents came to America from Sweden, Russia, Lithuania, and Mongolia. And when my brother had his genetics tested through a National Geographic program, we found that about 50 percent of our genes were of Spanish origin. So should we be eating dairy, reindeer, seafood, and lingonberries; or will we thrive on pierogies stuffed with potatoes, pumpernickel bread, sweet-and-sour cabbage, yak, and mushroom stew? What about the Mediterranean diet, since we're half Mediterranean?

Simplifying the Carb Question

> The most basic practical consideration that governs how to eat for our metabolic type is simple: Given the environment in which we live, does the combination of our genetics, our gut microbes, and the food we eat (plus other factors that have yet to be discovered) lead us to be (1) exquisitely insulin sensitive, (2) moderately insulin sensitive, or (3) insulin resistant? How can we know?

One way we can know is by our weight.

After an initial weight loss of five or six pounds on the ultra-low-fat, high-carb diet that was the starting point in our diet sleuthing, both Gordon and I started to gain weight back steadily. That's often the pattern when you change your diet. You lose some weight, and then over time you put it back on, perhaps with interest.

At the end of 14 months on a high-carb diet (even though it was high in fiber), I tipped the scale at 127 pounds—five pounds more than when I'd started the diet. At 5'3", that was my highest weight ever. Furthermore, the bonus pounds showed up in the worst part of the anatomy from a health standpoint: the belly.

Ravenously hungry most of the time, I got caught up in a carb-craving cycle that had me eating Ezekiel 4:9 bread toast before bed. Since the low-fat diet nixed butter, I ate the toast with organic raspberry jam—carbs on top of carbs. A slice of Ezekiel 4:9 bread has 12 net grams of carbs once you deduct the fiber. A half-table-spoon of jam adds another 7 grams. *Nineteen grams of carbs (and we're talking about a single piece of high-fiber toast with jam) is nearly a sixth of the 130 grams recommended by mainstream government agencies for both kids and adults.* No wonder I was piling on the pounds.

In the next Science Bite, we'll compare the carbs in an average day of eating a Standard American Diet (SAD) with a PlantPlus Diet day.

CHAPTER 17

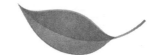

The SAD Truth and the PlantPlus Solution

"There's a lot of money in the Western diet. The more you process any food, the more profitable it becomes. The healthcare industry makes more money treating chronic diseases (which account for three quarters of the $2 trillion plus we spend each year on health care in this country) than preventing them."

— MICHAEL POLLAN

Consider this scenario. I'm giving a presentation at a psychology conference during the ultra-low-fat, high-carb phase of our diet experiment. As a traveling vegan eating out, this means consuming a lot of pasta and bread.

I head out to dinner with two other women. Our destination is a restaurant we've chosen because it features local, farm-to-table, whole-foods ingredients. One of the women is a vegetarian who is about 40 pounds overweight. The other is a sleek, muscular Paleo eater who orders a big steak with spinach and mushrooms and a side of asparagus. Tiny though she is—maybe a size 2—she puts away the whole thing. The chubby vegetarian and I dutifully eat our pasta, veggies, and bread.

There's no better way to get a handle on the difference between the high-carb, low-quality Standard American Diet (SAD) that you're leaving behind and the high-quality, carb-reasonable PlantPlus Diet that you're moving toward, than comparing the two head to head. So let's crunch a few numbers so that you can see why it's so easy to get chubby eating 350 grams of high-GI carbs every day.

An Average SAD Day in Carb Grams

Breakfast
Glass of OJ (8 ounces): 25 g. (basically liquid sugar)
Multigrain bagel: 69 g. (basically solid sugar)
2 Tbsp. real cream cheese or vegan substitute: 1 g.
1 Tbsp. commercial strawberry jam: 14 g. (basically sugar)
2 tsp. sugar in coffee: 10 g.
Total Carb Grams: 119

Snack: *Half* a fruit Danish (Oh, you're so good!): 24 g.

Lunch
Turkey (or tofu) sandwich on whole-grain bread: 54 g.
    Turkey: 3 ounces lean deli turkey breast: 12 g. (all from added sugar)
    Tofu: 0 g.
    Bread (2 slices): 42 g.
Small bag potato chips: 16 g.
Apple: 14 g.
2 Oreo cookies: 18 g.
Total Carb Grams: 93–105

Snack: Energy Bar (Cliff): 46 g.
or 12-ounce soda: 39 g.
Both: 85 g. (Good gravy!)

Dinner
Skinless chicken breast or a vegetable-based protein: 0 g.
Baked potato: 37 g.
Broccoli: 8 g.
½ cup lemon sorbet: 23 g.
½ cup fresh raspberries: 7 g.
Total Carb Grams: 75

This typical SAD day—three meals and two snacks—totals about 320 grams of carbs, give or take a few. In contrast—and yes, I know you know this, but repetition always helps—both the United States Department of Agriculture and the Institute of Medicine recommend just 130 grams of carbs per day for both adults and children.[1]

This SAD day is way over the limit.

An Average PlantPlus Day in Carb Grams

Even though I don't recommend counting carbs in low-starch veggies, I've done it here for comparison's sake.

Breakfast
2-egg very veggie omelet: 2–6 g.
1 cup cooked oatmeal (½ cup dry): 22 g.
2 thin slices almond-bread toast: 4 g.
½ cup blueberries: 10 g.

Total Carb Grams:
omnivore no-grain breakfast: 16 g.
vegan no-egg breakfast: 32 g.

Snack: one medium apple: 14 g.
And/or ¼ cup nuts: 7 g.

21 g. for both

Lunch

Huge green salad with assorted raw veggies including carrots, avocado, radish, cucumber, tomato, or whatever is handy: 2–6 g.

Protein source: Half a cup, could be cheese (feta = 3 g.), meat (negligible), eggs (1 g.), tofu (2 g.), or tempeh (8 g.) A whole cup of protein is not much more in terms of carbs.

Total Carb Grams: 10–12

Snack: 2 PlantPlus Cookies: 2–3 g.

Dinner

Savory stew of lamb and vegetables: 6–8 g. For vegans eating vegetarian chili: 35 g.
Chunk of almond bread: 7 g.
Salad: 5 g.
Glass of good red wine if you like, water with lemon, or plain old water: 0 g.
Berry-Cherry Gel-Yo: 5 g. (the recipe is in Part IV)

Total Carb Grams: 30ish for omnivores; 50ish for vegans

Daily Total: 90–100 grams for omnivores; about 140 for vegans

Hey, isn't this how we're supposed to be eating, at least in terms of carb grams?

A Note about Salt

I love salty food and snacks. But even though I use a little salt in my cooking, and shake a little more on my food, I still come in at about 1,500 mg/day on a PlantPlus Diet—the amount recommended for people with high blood pressure and cardiovascular disease, or those with African-American ancestry.

The average American on a SAD diet, on the other hand, eats more than 3,300 mg sodium daily. A relative who eats a lot of processed foods was upset by my use of the salt shaker until I pointed out that only 10 percent of sodium in a SAD diet comes from home cooking and the salt shaker. The remainder comes from processed foods and eating out in restaurants.

Here's the breakdown from the Centers for Disease Control (CDC), a government agency whose name is pretty self-explanatory. If you go to their website, you'll find the following revelatory facts about salt:[2]

- More than 75 percent of the sodium Americans consume comes from prepackaged, processed, and restaurant foods.

- A mere 5 percent of dietary sodium gets added in home cooking. Another 6 percent comes from salting food at the table.

- About 12 percent of sodium occurs naturally in whole foods.

- A lot of the packaged foods we eat are loaded with sodium but don't even taste salty.

- Breads and rolls, cold cuts, and pizza are the major sources of sodium in the American diet. (Okay, I get the cold cuts and even the pizza. But breads and rolls? You could have fooled me there.) The CDC reinforced the bread statistic by adding that a single slice of bread generally contains 80 to 230 mg of sodium.

- Two slices of bread eat up one-third of the recommended sodium allowance for about half the U.S. population ("People 51 and older and those of any age who are African Americans or who have high blood pressure, diabetes, or chronic kidney disease").

Let's revisit the apparently healthy turkey sandwich that so many Americans eat for lunch, taking a peak at the sodium content. I chose the products in the example as representative of what Americans buy in large-chain supermarkets.

Sodium in a Turkey Sandwich Lunch

Two slices of Safeway whole-wheat bread: 320 mg
One serving Kroger Deli Style Turkey Breast: 620 mg
Two Oreo cookies: 300 mg
One ounce Lay's Potato Chips: 154 mg
Small apple: 2 mg

Mg of sodium for lunch = 1,396

It's interesting that the potato chips, which might seem the saltiest item in the lunch, are actually the lowest in sodium, except for the apple. Considering that 1,500 mg per day is the sodium limit for half the population, it seems profligate to blow it all on a single meal. But since many of us don't read labels, we're not much concerned about all that sodium.

In a 2012 poll, about half the U.S. population (51.6 percent) paid attention to the list of ingredients on the label of a food product before purchasing it.[3] *The rest of us would be a lot healthier if we read labels as well. Aim to make that a practice. Anything you buy needs to be given the hairy eyeball first and rejected if it contains:*

- Refined carbs like flour and sugar (pick your battles; a few won't kill you once in a while)

- Bad fats: polyunsaturated oils, particularly cottonseed oil, and trans fats

- Significant salt

- GMOs

- Chemicals

Now that you're in the know about measuring sugar, fat, and salt in food, we'll turn our attention to measuring some important health markers in your own body. In the next chapter, I'll tell you about a few basic blood tests that can tell you where you're at metabolically. Are you insulin sensitive or insulin resistant? Knowing that is the key to motivation for better health. Those numbers will also help you tailor your PlantPlus lifestyle to your own metabolic needs.

CHAPTER 18

Checking Your Insulin Resistance:

What Tests to Ask For and Why

"My doctor gave me six months to live. But when I couldn't pay the bill, he gave me six months more."

— WALTER MATTHAU

Television ads for drugs abound. Ask your doctor if this drug or that is right for you! Try the little purple pills. Here's a great drug . . . and there are just a few side effects—like dropping dead. After we listen to the side effects of some of these drugs, usually reeled off while we watch a "patient" having the time of their life, it's a wonder that we still ask our doctors for a prescription for anything. But we do; otherwise, drug companies wouldn't be spending the money to educate consumers on what to ask for.

It's sad that we're turning our physicians into drug pushers. At the same time, these ads reflect the fact that the average person is becoming more interested in finding out medical facts and tracking down appropriate treatments for whatever might be ailing them.

But rather than closing the barn door after the horse is stolen—asking for a drug when you're already sick—it would be much better if we knew enough to ask for appropriate medical tests so that we could prevent illness in the first place. That's what this chapter is all about.

Basic Tests for Metabolism

If you don't know what your metabolism is like when you start a diet, you won't be able to tell if the diet is doing you good or killing you off. When Gordon had a lipid profile done after a year on the ultra-low-fat, high-carb diet we started our diet experimentation with, the results were shocking. Almost all his test results had gotten worse, rather than better. He had actually developed insulin resistance and metabolic syndrome. (Remember that one man's meat is another man's poison and that many people thrive on the same nutritional protocol that didn't work for us.)

So before you start messing with your food, it's wise to go to the doc and ask for some tests that can give you a reliable baseline for *your* diet experiment. The following simple blood tests will help you and your doc understand where you are on the insulin-sensitivity spectrum—the bell-shaped curve that we discussed in Chapter 16, "Going Carb-Reasonable." The more insulin resistant you are, the fewer carbs you need to eat. The good news is that even a month of eating more nutrient-dense, lower-GI foods can reduce insulin resistance and even reverse metabolic syndrome in some people.

Here are a few tests to ask for. Your doctor may suggest similar tests from other sources, plus tests I'm not covering here:

1. **NMR Lipid Profile.** LipoScience (www.liposcience.com) offers an NMR (nuclear magnetic resonance) lipid profile that evaluates blood lipids including LDL-C, HDL-C, and various other lipid categories including particle size and LDL-P (cholesterol particle

number, now thought to be a better measure of heart disease risk than either LDL concentration or particle size). The test correlates these measures with insulin resistance and diabetes risk. If your doc sends you to LabCorp (a national chain) for the test, make sure that LabCorp Test code #884000 is specified. While the test is not yet certified by the FDA, it's thought to be a good composite measure of insulin resistance. Your insulin sensitivity (the LP-IR score) is given as a percentile of a reference population, ranging from 0 (most insulin sensitive) to 100 (most insulin resistant). After I was on our PlantPlus, carb-reasonable diet for a few months, this test confirmed that I was highly insulin sensitive (13th percentile). Gordon was even more insulin sensitive, coming in at the 9th percentile. Unfortunately, since we didn't have this measure prior to starting on our carb-right lifestyle, we had no previous figures to compare it to. Since insulin resistance predisposes to developing cardiovascular disease over time, we're both happy that our IR levels are so low. We'll continue to track them.

2. **HbA1c.** If you have diabetes, your doc already tracks your blood level of glycated hemoglobin (HbA1c) regularly, every three to six months. HbA1c is a measure of your average blood-glucose levels for the previous two to three months. If blood sugar is high, it sticks to the hemoglobin molecules inside the red blood cells through the process called *glycation* that you're already familiar with. Because red blood cells live anywhere from 6 to 12 weeks, HbA1c is an average measure of blood sugar during that time. The normal range is about 5 percent. Prediabetes is diagnosed between 5.7 and 6.4 percent. At 6.5 percent and above, diabetes is diagnosed.[1]

3. **Cardioreactive Protein (C-reactive protein or CRP)** is a common marker for general inflammation, also used as a marker for cardiovascular disease risk. Because CRP rises rapidly when you have an infection, a burn, or other trauma, this test should be done when you're feeling well. Low risk: less than 1.0 mg/L; Average risk: 1.0 to 3.0 mg/L; High risk: 3.0 mg/L or above.

4. Fasting Plasma Glucose (FPG) is a measure of how much glucose is in your blood after you've been fasting for at least eight hours. Caffeine can change the results, so skip the coffee or tea the morning of your blood test. A fasting range of 70–99 mg/dL is considered normal. Prediabetic levels range from 100–125. Diabetes is diagnosed at 126 or above.

5. Fasting Insulin Level: Normal levels of circulating insulin are less than 10 µU/mL. You're at risk for diabetes when the level rises to 10–12 µU/mL. Diabetes is generally diagnosed at levels above 12 µU/mL, using a reference range of 3–25 µU/mL.

Low-carb diets are popular because, as you know, they're the best way to lose weight and keep it off (that is, if you eat a lot of vegetables). The reason that these diets are successful, at least in part, is because they lower insulin resistance.

No matter whose low-carb diet formula you follow—whether it's *The New Atkins for a New You*, cardiologist William Davis's *Wheat Belly* program, cardiologist Arthur Agatston's *South Beach Diet*, nutritionist Jonny Bowden's *Living the Low Carb Life*, heart surgeon Steven Gundry's *Diet Evolution*, neurologist David Perlmutter's *Grain Brain* diet, any of the Paleo-type diets, or books written by women gynecologists like Sara Gottfried's *The Hormone Cure* or Diana Schwarzbein's *The Schwarzbein Principle*—you'll most likely see four changes in your blood lipids if they were high to begin with:

1. Your triglycerides will decline markedly.

2. Your HDL, or good cholesterol, will go up.

3. Your LDL, or bad cholesterol, may either go up, down, or stay the same. Since opinions on whether or not LDL concentration per se makes any difference at all to heart disease are controversial and change every few months, right now this isn't the most important benchmark of how diet affects cardiovascular disease (CVD) risk.

4. The particle size of your LDL (which is now thought to be more important than total cholesterol concentration in blood, or LDL-C) will convert to large and fluffy (Pattern A), which is relatively heart healthy as opposed to the small atherogenic Pattern B. Particle size is generally concordant with LDL-P or total particle number. But don't get complacent just because you've got large particles. Some people with large particles still have high particle number, elevating risk for CVD. There are several reasons why that can happen, including genetic proclivity. If that's true of you, your doc will need to monitor LDL-P carefully as you change your diet.

Congratulations!

You have now eaten all or hopefully most of the Science Bites that serve as a foundation for how to eat right for your metabolism and why. There are many more fine points, of course, but my aim has been to paint a big picture for you. You can review the Science Bites whenever the craving strikes, and over time you'll digest them and make this fascinating material an integral part of who you are.

In Part II of this book—coming right up—we'll turn our attention to lifestyle issues. This is where the fun really starts. While as a cell biologist I love the science, as a pleasure-oriented human being, I'm motivated by a delicious PlantPlus lifestyle.

And as a licensed psychologist, I'm fascinated with how our mind, emotions, and sensibilities can either help us change our lives for the better or put up roadblocks that keep us stuck. My hope in Part II is to take down the roadblocks so that you can cruise happily into a delicious, healthful PlantPlus lifestyle.

PART II

LIFESTYLE
BITES

Now that you've read some Science Bites (you can always go back for seconds), we'll start the practical part of your journey to a PlantPlus life with the information you need to put the science into practice.

In the last section, we discussed medical tests to help you discover the diet right for your metabolism. In this section, we'll discuss your own perceptions and reflections as guides. Then you'll enter the gates of food heaven with a preview of the delights in store for you. Next we'll move on to the fascinating world of neuroscience and mindfulness. You'll learn the art of how to train your brain for food success. Food cravings often sabotage even the most heartfelt desire for change, so I want you to know exactly how to outwit them. The final chapter in this section is the last preparatory step before you begin the PlantPlus Reboot process in Part III. It's all about clearing out the old to make room for the new.

Here we go, fellow travelers. Buckle up for a trip to pleasure and fun!

CHAPTER 19

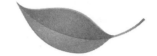

Self-Knowledge:

Your New Life as a Lab Rat

"He who knows others is learned;
He who knows himself is wise."

— LAO-TZU, TAO TE CHING

What? Being a lab rat is not your idea of food heaven? Be patient, and we'll enter the realm of a delicious lifestyle in the next chapter. But before we do that, we need to start where we are.

The first step in any journey is to look around. We look back to see where we came from and at the ground we're standing on to appreciate where we are. This pause in order to reflect helps us lock on to the vision of where we want to go.

The journey to health through personalized nutrition is no exception. By the time Gordon and I got serious about finding a diet that our bodies could thrive on, we were in our 60s. The boundless energy of youth was starting to fade, and the chronic illnesses of aging were gradually staking a claim to our lives.

This unhappy state of affairs had a bright side: It was a wake-up call that gave us a new vision. What we really wanted was to enjoy this precious life for as long as possible, in roadworthy physical vehicles.

The vision of renewed vitality required some serious self-reflection. In the last chapter, we considered some lab tests that provide a compass to guide the healing journey. In this chapter, we'll look at self-tests that add another level of self-knowledge to the process of diet personalization and renewed health.

> A good motto for this journey of discovery is the following: *Know thyself, feed thyself, heal thyself, and, most of all . . . enjoy thyself.*

Reflecting on Your Diet History

My own retrospection included harvesting the wisdom of 40 years of diet sleuthing. A vegetarian in my late 20s and early 30s, I had to stop when I became so wan and thin that a rumor circulated around the medical school where I taught that I had leukemia. In spite of eating practically anything I could lay my hands on, my weight dropped to an anorexic-looking 99 pounds.

Brought to my senses by the rumor, I reluctantly added chicken and fish to my whole-foods diet. That adjustment improved my health and energy dramatically. Since I'd been a careful vegetarian, supplementing with vitamin B_{12} and combining foods with different amino acids to make complete proteins, I didn't understand why my health suffered so badly. I still don't, but when Gordon and I were first diagnosed with heart disease, I reasoned that many years had passed and that perhaps my body had changed to the point where a vegetarian or vegan diet might work for me.

Unfortunately, as you already know, it didn't.

When my health and Gordon's, too, went down the tubes after 14 months on what we affectionately termed the "hair-shirt diet" (because going fat-free felt so much like doing penance), we knew that something had to change—and quickly. I needed to get my newly virulent diet-related hypertension under control, and Gordon needed to reverse his brand-new carb-induced lipid abnormalities.

We were sitting at the kitchen counter one day—eating a lunch of grilled tofu on Ezekiel 4:9 bread with lettuce, tomato, and grilled onions—when I explained to Gordon where my scientific fact-seeking had led. I suggested that we make a complete lifestyle turnaround to a PlantPlus, vegetable-rich, carb-reasonable diet with plenty of protein and good fat, starting with a grass-fed ribeye steak for dinner.

Gordon turned as white as a sheet.

Just ten minutes previously, he, like most of the medical establishment, had thought of fat as the mortal enemy. Gordon's cardiologist reacted to his decision to try a low-carb diet with some skepticism. "You're going low carb? No grain? That's Paleo," she observed, clearly concerned. She was worried that eating a diet that included meat might cause inflammation, a serious underlying factor in the genesis of coronary artery disease.

Well, technically, we weren't planning to eat a Paleo diet. Even though long-term studies are lacking, it does appear to work well for some people. Academic nutritionists, however, are not generally among those in favor. The Paleo diet was rated dead-last out of 29 diets by an expert panel charged with reviewing the research for *U.S. News* and telling us what we should be eating.[1] The panel members might try their own diet sleuthing. Perhaps they'd come to a different conclusion. Perhaps not.

Fortunately, we had some baseline data with which to evaluate our diet change, including lab tests for inflammation. The results of all our previous lab tests—plus weight, blood-pressure readings, and evaluating our mood—provided a solid basis for the new diet experiment. After several weeks on PlantPlus, Gordon had his lab tests repeated. There was no problem with inflammation, thankfully. His CRP level (an indicator of inflammation, as we discussed in the last chapter) had dropped to nearly zero. My blood pressure also dropped, and the weight we'd both gained from eating so many carbs melted away.

> If you're changing your diet because of a health problem, you need to be a good lab rat, too, making sure that health measures are improving rather than worsening.

Keeping Track of How You Feel

There's no room for wishful thinking or diet zealotry in your personal laboratory of discovery. If I hadn't kept a diary of changes in mood and health for the first three months of our PlantPlus experiment, I might have missed some very important changes: no more achy, arthritic hips that made sleeping a nightmare; a complexion that was clear and luminous; increased stress hardiness and mood stability; a brighter attitude; moist skin instead of alligator hide; shiny hair rather than witchy locks; and the disappearance of migraine headaches.

No, I'm not exaggerating. It's hard to remember how you felt yesterday or the day before—let alone weeks or months before—unless you track your physical symptoms in an organized fashion. For that reason, I've included a Medical Symptom Checklist (MSCL) in the Appendix for you to fill out. This simple checklist was designed and validated (meaning that it works reliably) by Jane Leserman, Ph.D., a colleague of mine from my Harvard days and an expert in research design and statistics. The MSCL takes only a few minutes to fill out and provides a reliable baseline so that when you fill it out again after four weeks on your new diet, you can tell whether you're improving or not.

Open Mind, Open Mouth

It wasn't easy to change our diet from vegan to omnivore. We were eating low on the food chain and helping the planet. We were practicing kindness to animals. All true, of course, and this is the reason why many people choose to be vegans or vegetarians: as a matter of conscience. I applaud you if you've made that choice, and hope that the information in this book will help you stay with it in a way that's most beneficial for you.

But Gordon and I had to keep to our primary vision—getting healthy again—even though it meant consuming animal products.

Once we adjusted our attitude to one of omnivorous open-mindedness, we scoured the pantry, the fridge, and the freezer for the carbs that were causing health problems. We collected two entire cartons of whole-wheat and brown-rice pasta, quinoa and brown rice, amaranth and barley, oatmeal and seven-grain cereal, organic cold cereals, sprouted whole-grain breads, low-fat granola, whole-grain English muffins, rice cakes, potatoes, whole-grain crackers, raw sugar, honey, maple syrup, jams, jellies, agave nectar, ketchup, and sugar-rich marinades.

It was fun giving away the food to friends, many of whom thought we'd lost our ever-lovin' minds. Another diet? And this one a 180-degree about-face from the one we'd been on for 14 months and defended with such zealous vigor? First, no fat and mostly veggies, fruits, and grains; and now, fat is okay, but grains are bad?

I learned quite a bit about the results of our dietary change from keeping a food and blood-pressure log. I could have learned even more by organizing my reflections, so I've laid out a simple way to do that (you'll get to the Daily Diet Reflections in a moment) to make your journey a little bit easier. Your informal daily reflections don't replace the MSCL; rather, they're a personal, ongoing addition that keep you informed of and motivated by your progress. If something needs to change, you'll recognize that sooner rather than later.

I kept notes on a computer, but it might be even easier to buy an inexpensive spiral notebook and use one page for each day, remembering to date your entries so that you can make sense of your results over time.

Daily Diet Reflections

- What did you eat? By keeping track, you can start to notice patterns. For example, foods that make you gassy, keep you up at night, make you achy, create allergic symptoms, and so forth.

- Was your sleep restful, or not?

- How do you feel physically?

- Any changes in weight, blood pressure, blood glucose, or any other measures you routinely track?

- What was your mood like?

- What was your energy like?

- Jot down any other observations you think are important. Having enough energy to hike up the mountain where we were living at 9,000 feet was a big one for me, as was the excitement of trying on a beloved pair of 30-year-old cutoffs that finally fit again. While positive observations are vital for staying motivated, negative observations are just as significant because they highlight foods that may be problematic.

Now that we've covered the importance of documenting where you start out so that you can appreciate the changes along the way, we'll dive into the nitty-gritty of the PlantPlus lifestyle in the next chapter. But first, a few tips on launching the journey of a lifetime.

Tips for Launching a PlantPlus Lifestyle

1. Call a meeting to discuss why you want to eat the PlantPlus way with everyone in your household. When people feel seen and heard, and are confident that their opinion counts, your household will feel more harmonious and cooperative. Eating whole foods and eliminating processed food is a bottom line for all family members that you'll need to negotiate.

2. Another issue to discuss is that Plus foods vary depending on metabolic needs, values, and preferences. Perhaps one family member is a vegetarian, for example, and believes that everyone should eat in the same way, but someone else in the household thrives on animal protein. *Judging others' Plus foods and trying to convert them to yours is a no-no.*

3. As adults we're capable of making our own choices. Children, however, are not. If they're used to eating processed foods, sweets, and pasta all the time, there's going to be an adjustment to eating whole foods. Don't worry—it can be done. I liked Mee Tracy McCormick's discussion of how to switch kids to a whole-foods diet in her delightful book, *My Kitchen Cure*. They eat "Mee-ified" food at home but can still eat some of their old favorites outside the house.

4. Fill out the Medical Symptom Checklist (MSCL), which you'll find in the Appendix. Make two copies, since you'll be filling it out again in four weeks. Keep your MSCL in a safe place so that you'll be able to refer back to it as a baseline for your progress. Without a health record, you'd be guessing about how you felt a day ago, let alone a month ago. The results of your MSCL will help you personalize your

diet after the Reboot, an art that we'll address in Chapter 23.

5. Make an appointment for a medical checkup, and ask for the tests in the previous chapter. A baseline measure of your blood lipids, blood pressure, fasting insulin, fasting glucose, HbA1c, and your insulin-resistance score will help you see where you currently stand, where you need to go, and whether—after the four-week PlantPlus Reboot—you're actually getting there. If your doc is curious and up-to-date, you'll make a good diet-sleuthing team.

That's it, folks. You're almost ready to launch your new Plant-Plus lifestyle. But first, a necessary motivational pep talk in the next chapter. You're not going to dietary hell. I promise. In fact, the gates of food heaven are about to open before you.

CHAPTER 20

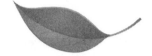

PlantPlus Diet Heaven

"I cook with wine. Sometimes I even add it to the food."

— W.C. FIELDS

I've always dreaded the word *diet*. It calls up images of penance, misery, hunger, and food that tastes like cardboard or swine slop. It's like going to jail. On the other hand, you may have images of people who go overboard with their views on healthy eating and carry on like humorless religious zealots bound on making you feel like a sinner. Jokes about the indignities of health food, after all, are the stock-in-trade of comedians.

I've said it before, and I'll say it again: The PlantPlus Diet isn't a diet in the traditional sense—it's a lifestyle that you're going to love.

Take a moment now to pretend that you can reach into your brain and pull out all your images of what eating healthy is like. If some of them still work for you after reading this chapter, then you can put them back in. In the meantime, let's install a different set of images into that smart brain of yours.

> You are not going to food hell. In fact, you are about to become the creator of food heaven, right in your own kitchen.

But first, let's take a trip to the market.

One of the most enjoyable parts of traveling to places like India, Egypt, Turkey, Mexico, or Peru are the open-air markets. They're a lively riot of colorful produce, spices, cheeses, meats, medicinal herbs, shamanic supplies, animated merchants, haggling shoppers, donkeys and carts, trucks and buses, the occasional camel, and the fragrant aromas of street-food cooking. Do I eat those local delicacies? Generally not, since the microbes in those parts of the world are foreign to my American-grown tummy. But Gordon and I did survive a delicious lunch of delicate roast pigeon in the famed Khan el-Khalili marketplace in Cairo.

It was culinary heaven and a delight for all the senses. Even if your farmer's market is lacking in camels or shamans, you can still have a really good time there.

The Fun and Integrity of the Market

Here in the United States, open-air markets, where local farmers sell their marvelous dirt- and microbe-encrusted wares, are making a comeback. They're a far cry from shopping for processed food in the decidedly unnatural environments of Walmart, Target, and chain supermarkets.

The food at a real farmers' market is fresh and alive. You can ask questions about who grew it and what its life was like. Did those eggs come from happy hens or debeaked prisoners languishing in a cage? Is that coffee or chocolate fair trade? Were the laborers paid enough to feed their own families?

A PlantPlus lifestyle honors the journey that whole foods make from the earth to your lips. Before you engage in an act as physically and emotionally intimate as eating—taking food into your body and inviting it to become part of you—it's wise to ask if the food has integrity. Are those greens organic and fresh? Is the salmon Atlantic (a code for *farm raised*) or wild caught? Is that corn a natural grain or a GMO? Living with mindful, respectful awareness of the whole is what makes a PlantPlus Diet into a PlantPlus Diet Solution that improves the quality of life all around.

When you eat the PlantPlus way, you help family farms survive and do well by doing good. You become a steward of the Earth, protecting it from pesticides, herbicides, and untested agricultural practices like the unprecedented genetic gamble on GMOs. You help the animals that give their lives as food enjoy a good life in their time. Your choice of fair-trade products helps ensure that farmworkers can earn a living wage. And, of course, by living a PlantPlus lifestyle, you become a champion of your own health and that of your family's.

A PlantPlus Feast

Okay, I kept my "PlantPlus Lifestyle Solution" stump speech short.

The rest of what I have to say about a PlantPlus Diet lifestyle is really simple. It's easy to prepare, incredibly enjoyable, and may surprise you by igniting a new passion for cooking. Preparing real food can be a wonderful solitary, contemplative activity. It's also a great way to spend time with family and friends.

We asked David and Chris, friends of many years—what we call *family by choice*—to our home for dinner one New Year's Eve. I'd set the table with thick, hand-painted pottery plates and Mexican-style blue-rimmed glasses. The table looked gracious and inviting, both before dinner and after . . . since we never did get around to sitting down there.

All four of us were perched on stools around the kitchen island chopping veggies, so we put out hors d'oeuvres in our workspace. Gordon brought out his signature guacamole and a festive plate of sliced jicama, carrots, and celery. I added a plate of the tasty toasted-sesame crackers that I made out of almond flour. Then along came some nutty and delicious sheep's milk cheese and a bowl of big, fresh blueberries.

The topic of conversation turned to conservation, so I produced a bar of my favorite Alter Eco dark chocolate. It's a fair-trade chocolate made from the beans of cacao trees that have reforested the land and replaced cocaine as the main income source in the area of Ecuador where they're grown. The farmers can now make a living and be free from the dangerous drug trade in which they were previously expendable pawns.

Everyone tried a square of the 70 percent dark-chocolate almond bar. If you let small bits of it melt in your mouth, a single square lasts for a long time. An added benefit was how well the chocolate went with the healthful and delicious red wine we were drinking. It would have gone just as well with sparkling water, in case alcohol isn't right for you. But we did feel like kings and queens, savoring all the little plates in front of us as we continued to talk and chop vegetables for the main course.

Next (remember that this was a festive meal and far richer than usual) came another appetizer: organic, free-range chicken wings roasted crispy after a brief toss in olive oil, fresh chili powder, and herbs. Then came the kale, fennel, apple, and sunflower-seed salad that I'd made in advance that afternoon (the recipes for this meal are in Part IV). We also put out a bowl of the tangy, probiotic sauerkraut that we'd recently finished fermenting.

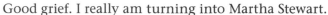

Good grief. I really am turning into Martha Stewart.

Then the fragrance of roasted sweet potatoes flooded the kitchen. Still sitting around the island with our guests, we scooped the potatoes out of their jackets, which we saved for our big standard poodles, Milo and Mitzi. Sweet potatoes are naturally sweet, and ours need just a hint of butter and a little salt and pepper to bring out their mouthwatering flavor.

Our friend Chris was in charge of chopping the *mirepoix*. I learned that somewhat daunting French word from a Cajun swamp guide who taught me that a trio of finely chopped carrots, celery, and onions—combined with some cracker crumbs and chicken or veggie stock—makes the perfect stuffing for seafood. He wasn't kidding. The stuffed shrimp we made for the main course was the best thing I ever ate.

Our original plan for a sit-down dinner turned into a three-hour feast of tapas—small dishes, a style popular in Mediterranean countries. Serving a meal dish-by-dish as it's ready, rather than having to coordinate an "upstairs" feast with no "downstairs" help, allowed Gordon and me to avoid a whole lot of stress that night. We enjoyed the meal as thoroughly, as did our guests.

I travel about a third of the time, giving lectures and workshops across the country, so relaxing at home isn't just a ho-hum event. It's as necessary for maintaining my sanity as breathing clean air or drinking fresh water. The kitchen is what calls, offering sanctuary and a way to root back into home.

> Our streamlined, well-organized PlantPlus kitchen is a playground for creativity—a lifestyle laboratory where we can try new things and take some risks. Once in a while, a new dish fails miserably, but that is a good thing since it's always instructive.

Cooking at home is the most cost-effective way to eat well and have a lot of fun doing it. While some of the ingredients in our special New Year's Eve dinner were a bit pricey, most of them were not. And a restaurant meal would have cost a whole lot more. Furthermore, the leftovers were divine. Gordon and I sat down at our unused, elegant table on New Year's Day and made a brunch out of whatever was left from the night before.

It's strange to say, but one of the most unexpected delights of going to food heaven turns out to be leftovers. Eating them is like going to a restaurant, since there are no pots and pans to clean up after the feast you've already prepared.

Changing Your Mind

I hope that our short visit to PlantPlus heaven has opened your mind to the glorious lifestyle that awaits you. I also hope that whatever images of food hell that may have lurked in your neural circuitry, before our tour of markets and feasts, are now gone. If you did the little exercise that I suggested at the beginning of the chapter—reaching into your brain and taking out all the images you have about healthy eating—perhaps there are now some really heavenly images in your mind's eye. In that case, take a minute and put them back in.

In the next chapter, we're doing more than imagining a reprogramming of your brain. I'm going to put on my Psychologist's Hat (a black felt cowboy hat) and tell you how to rewire your brain to avoid food cravings so that you can live a happy PlantPlus lifestyle evermore.

CHAPTER 21

Rewiring Your Brain to Reduce Cravings and Enhance Pleasure

"Every man can, if he so desires, become
the sculptor of his own brain."

— Neuroscientist Santiago Ramón y Cajal

A happy lifestyle of any kind involves two things: First, you have to identify and remove any roadblocks that get in the way of your progress—in this case, it is cravings for highly rewarding but health-sabotaging, junk food. Second, you need to focus your intention on having fun and feeling pleasure while you're moving toward the goal—*PlantPlus Food Heaven.*

If you're not having fun, whatever you're doing will begin to feel stale, and you'll eventually give it up. The point of this chapter is to remove some of the roadblocks to attaining food heaven and rewire your brain to appreciate the journey with more mindful, highly motivating pleasure. This isn't just psychobabble, by the way. It's neuroscience. I'd bet my cowboy hat on it.

Neuroplasticity

The big news in science that predated sequencing the human genome, and the discovery that we are more microbe than mammal, concerns the brain. It's not a done deal. We used to think that the brain we were born with lost some of its cells as we aged (it does), but that it didn't have the capacity to form new connections and rewire itself (it does). This revolution in thinking is called *neuroplasticity*.

Neuroplasticity is important because it's the basis of learning. Think about how water runs down a mountain: It rains and rivulets form. The rivulets coalesce into streams, and the streams feed into a river. Every time it rains, water runs in the same course. The brain works in the same way. But with neuroplasticity, we can form new rivulets and divert the flow of water—neural activity— into new pathways. Old dogs can definitely learn new tricks. We can change behaviors—even ingrained eating behaviors—by changing brain circuitry.

Here's the truth that all of us have to deal with when we adapt to a new dietary way of life: *It's hard.* We miss the old foods. Cravings can and will come along, especially early in a diet change before your brain has had the chance to create new wiring. The Reboot phase of the PlantPlus Diet that you'll read about in Part III lasts for 28 days, long enough for new neural pathways to form. Before you start, it's important for us to examine a few simple ways to use neuroplasticity to prevent cravings and keep your PlantPlus Reboot on track.

Maybe you're in the coffee shop ordering a latte, and your eyes light upon—*Oh God, give me strength*—a big, squishy, fragrant cinnamon bun. The saliva starts to collect in the back of your mouth. Before you know it, you've given in and that bun is now yours. Well, what the hell; it's just once in a while. The problem with eating that bun, however—especially during the Reboot—is that you're setting yourself up for failure and continued cravings. Let me explain why.

The Mysteries of Operant Conditioning

During college, I hung out in the rat room. No, I don't mean my boyfriend's dorm room—I mean the psych lab. For two hours a day, six days a week, I put rats (as well as pigeons, goldfish, and turtles) through their paces. We were studying how animals learn.

Both as an undergraduate at Bryn Mawr College and as a doctoral student at Harvard Medical School, I conducted experiments with a kind of learning called *operant conditioning*. What's that? An animal (remember that we're animals, too) performs some behavior— a rat presses a lever, for example—and the behavior causes a food pellet to drop into a dispenser. Every time the rat presses the lever, he gets a reward. This is called *continuous reinforcement.*

If you stop giving the rat rewards, however, he'll cut his losses and give up lever-pressing very quickly. But if the rat is rewarded just once in a while on what's called a *variable-interval schedule of reinforcement* (that is, randomly, for instance, after every four lever presses, or after every 7, 40, 13, and so on), something fascinating happens.

The lever-pressing behavior becomes almost impossible to extinguish. The rodents keep looking for the goodies, pressing that lever with hopeful fervor, long after it has stopped raining pellets.

I'm guilty of anthropomorphizing here, but the rat is now in a continuous state of craving just like you might be in if you're used to buying yourself treats at the store once in a while.

Time for a true confession: My treat for entering a supermarket was once a stop at the bakery counter where I'd get a sugar-glazed doughnut to munch on while shopping. Yes, I know that you're supposed to pay for it first, but cravings tend to erode one's morals. I did pay for it eventually by presenting the empty bag to the checkout clerk.

> So what's the moral of the "rat and the Joanie" story? If you start to cheat once in a while—especially during the Reboot when you're developing new neural circuitry to support a different way of life—you're setting yourself up for continued cravings.

Avoid the hazard of putting yourself on a variable-interval reinforcement schedule by not bringing foods into the house that aren't on the menu. If you do, you're likely to have a nibble, put them away, sneak another nibble, and so forth. You'll keep craving the foods you're addicted to not because of anything conscious, not because of emotional eating, and not because you lack willpower, but simply because your brain has created a circuit of long-lasting expectation based on a variable-interval schedule of reinforcement.

This is one reason why you'll do better adopting a PlantPlus lifestyle if the other people in your household agree to quit eating junk food at home. If they want to eat it, please request that they do so out of the house. It's so disheartening to be good all day, only to come home and succumb to a stale box of Cap'n Crunch.

Although Gordon and I have been eating PlantPlus for a long time, we still don't keep carb-rich foods in the cupboard with a few exceptions: honey for sore throats, and sugar for guests' use and the hummingbird feeder.

> The bottom line for the Reboot is clear: *Do not cheat at all—either at home or when you go out—during these four weeks.* Cheating not only leads to continued cravings but also defeats the purpose of your food experiment, which is to weed out foods that cause physical and emotional problems. Later, after you know what foods suit your body best, you can indulge *occasionally* in things that are off the menu, but *keep indulgences out of the house.*

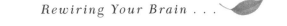

Ancient Brain, Modern Food Environment

Operant conditioning creates new brain circuits. Fortunately, you now know how to avoid wiring the brain to reinforce cravings. But what about ancient, already-wired brain circuits that make you superhungry when you lose weight? *Yikes! A famine,* the brain thinks. You better eat like mad when food becomes available so that you won't weaken and end your days as lion chow.

Because of this ancient survival circuit, slow weight loss, rather than starving to drop pounds in a hurry, is a more successful strategy for long-term success. Neuroscientist Sandra Aamodt points out that starvation has been a much more common problem than obesity in the history of human evolution. In the old hunter-gatherer days, if we starved in a famine, we needed to fatten up as soon as food became available. The brain's strategy for keeping us alive after a famine is twofold: First, as you already know, starvation makes you hungry so that you'll eat more food when you can get it. Second, your muscles compensate by burning less energy (which means using up fewer calories).

Aamodt made a stunning (and depressing) point in a June 2013 TED talk. People who lose weight need to reduce their caloric intake *forever* to keep it off. Your friend who weighs exactly the same as you do at your new weight, but didn't diet to get there, can eat a few hundred more calories every day.

As Aamodt reflects wistfully, no—life is *not* fair. None of her personal attempts at dieting, which had been ongoing since age 13, had worked—a fact that led her to find a way to outsmart the brain's old circuits. She's quite svelte now, which she attributes not to dieting, but to a slow weight loss through *mindful eating*. She eats when she's hungry and stops when she's full. I bet you're thinking, *Get real; that's not so easy.* Well, she did mention that it took her a year to figure out her body's signals so that she could become more aware of what her metabolism was telling her.

The problem in modern times is that if you drop weight fast, there's food everywhere to refeed upon. The sheer amount and variety of junk food on offer can defeat mindfulness. Think about it: There's junk food on display just about at every turn—from the hardware store to the Laundromat. Your ancient, postfamine brain circuits are constantly triggered by our modern, food-rich environment.

So how do you avoid succumbing to the old survival circuits?

One way is to be prepared with good snacks both at home and when you're out and about so that food and food ads don't send you running for the tortilla chips. I always keep nuts and an apple in the car to avoid being tempted by junk food at checkout counters. A few nuts can also provide safe passage through a movie to prevent you from giving in to a tub of greasy popcorn or a box of jelly beans.

But if you do, mindfulness of your inner dialogue can save you from falling down the rabbit hole and abandoning your new way of eating due to what psychologists call the *What-the-Hell Effect*.

Really, they do.

What the Hell Is the What-the-Hell Effect?

It's Thanksgiving, and you eat a piece of pumpkin pie. It's not normally on your diet, so you start to berate yourself. *Damn, I just blew my diet after all these weeks [or months]. I shouldn't have eaten that piece of pie. The crust is full of gluten [or calories or sugar, or it's processed, whatever]. I probably just gained a pound.*

As soon as you start talking to yourself like that, your inner saboteur opens the floodgates to eating more: *Well, I already ruined my diet, so I might as well have another piece of that pie.* So you eat a second piece of pie, which may not even have tasted so great in the first place, and now your inner saboteur goes into high gear.

Oh boy. I've really blown it now. I can't believe I just ate two pieces of that lousy pie. It wasn't even that good! But those chocolate truffles really do look good. What the hell . . . I've already made a mess of things, so I might as well have a couple of truffles. I love the ones with caramel and salt. . . .

The next morning you wake up feeling guilty. And when you go to the store, that doughnut you spot looks mighty good, so you say, "What the hell! You gotta live a little." And that, dear reader, is the beginning of the end. You judge yourself, are found wanting, and the emotional misery of failure leads to the catch-22 of mindless eating: You eat to feel better but end up feeling worse, which leads to eating more, which makes you feel worse . . . and the beat goes on while the pounds pile up. Self-judgment never leads to any place worth going.

Sandra Aamodt used mindfulness to pay close attention to what her body was telling her to eat and when. You can also use mindfulness to head off emotional eating at the pass and really enjoy the food that you do eat. You can find practical information about how to cultivate mindfulness in my *New York Times* bestseller *Minding the Body, Mending the Mind*. We'll do a few mindfulness exercises at the end of this chapter, as well. But for now, let's take a brief look at how mindfulness can prevent the activation of old brain circuits associated with self-judgment and create new brain circuits that hum with pleasure.

The Gift of Mindful Awareness

Consider this scenario: You're in the shower when some cue—your chubby belly, for instance—sends a signal to your brain. The sight of the flab activates your self-judgment circuit, and you say the same old stuff that you usually say about your physique. *Ugh, look at that belly. What a tub of lard. And that Science Bite on metabolic syndrome didn't help either. Now I know it's churning out pro-inflammatory cytokines. Maybe I'm even prediabetic. I hate myself!*

By the time you get out of the shower, you feel terrible. Maybe a cookie or two would help? You eat the cookie, catch another glimpse of the belly, and emotional eating has its way with you.

> Mindfulness is a mental stance and a brain-training practice that interrupts this unconscious emotional cycle. It clears away the roadblock of old neural circuitry and installs new wiring.

How does it do that, and what is *mindfulness* anyway?

Mindfulness is the ability to pay attention to what's actually happening in our moment-to-moment experience with curiosity and openness instead of judgment. Rather than getting swept away by the emotions (these arise from the survival circuitry in the midbrain), mindfulness switches brain activity to the *prefrontal cortex* (PFC), which is located behind the forehead and eyes. It's the part of the brain that can plan and carry out the necessary activities required to reach goals. The PFC is the most evolutionary-recent part of the brain. It gives us the gift (often experienced as a curse) of *self-awareness*.

Mindfulness is the latest word in stress reduction, law, medicine, business, education . . . you name it. That's no surprise because it's actually a form of brain hygiene that allows us to make choices more in keeping with our long-term goals than our momentary desires.

Okay, what the hell. So you ate all that pie. Let's switch gears from the repetitive, obnoxious self-talk that leads to emotional eating and practice mindfulness instead. How will we do that? Read through and try the two simple exercises in the following section.

Mindfulness Exercise to Reduce Craving

This simple exercise shifts brain activity from the emotional centers in the midbrain to the prefrontal cortex (PFC), the self-aware part of the brain that witnesses your thoughts. When you notice that your thinking is habitual and misery making ("stinkin' thinkin'"), this exercise can help you build up the mental muscles to *stop it*. Why let yourself go to a place with no redeeming value?

This exercise also stimulates neurosecretory cells (they make neurohormones that activate or inhibit brain circuitry) in the PFC. Cells in the middle of the PFC between your eyes release a hormone called gamma-aminobutyric acid (GABA), which inhibits the cells in your amygdala (an emotional center) from firing. In this way, the PFC activates your brain's built-in calming circuitry.

Breathing exercises like the one I'm about to teach you also change the rate of firing in an important nerve—the vagus nerve—one branch of which stimulates the heart. By increasing what's called *heart-rate variability* (HRV), which is beyond the scope of our discussion, increased vagal tone decreases cravings. When heart-rate variability is low, people who are addicted to substances or processes such as eating are more likely to indulge.

Our goal with this mindful-breathing exercise is to *increase* your HRV, *increase* GABA production, *shift brain activity* from the emotional centers to the prefrontal cortex, and help you either *pass up that second piece of pie* or at least *stop your habitual litany of self-judgment* if you do eat it. Here goes:

1. **Breathe in slowly through your nose**, just noticing the sensation of the air—perhaps its coolness as it enters your nostrils and anything else that you perceive about it. It doesn't matter *what* you notice, only *that* you notice. This is an awareness exercise.

2. **Purse your lips, and breathe out slowly**, as if you were breathing through a straw. Once again, pay close attention to the actual *sensation* of breathing. The slowed out-breath will reduce your breathing rate.

3. **Take four to eight of these mindful in-and-out breaths.**

4. **Return to the moment.** Notice how you feel. Maybe you feel more relaxed. Maybe your nose is itchy. Maybe you notice that colors are more vibrant.

Maybe your belt is tight. It doesn't matter. There's no good or bad here. After all, how we feel changes moment to moment. All that matters is that you're present and paying attention to the here and now, which is what mindfulness is all about. Mindfulness trains the brain to identify less with how you feel and more with the part of you that *witnesses* how you feel—the part of you that is self-aware. What part of the brain might that reside in? You remembered right if you said . . . the prefrontal cortex.

5. **Focus on more reasonable self-talk**, if you're still thinking about the pie, that is. You may be more interested in other things by now. But if you're still stuck in Pie Land, you might say, "I ate all that pie? Okay, it's not the end of the world. Maybe I'll take a few squares of dark chocolate along to the next holiday dinner and eat that instead of cruising the dessert table. Or maybe I'll eat half a piece of pie slowly, paying attention to the taste, the texture, and the feeling of the pie on my tastebuds. When I pay attention to what I'm eating, there's a lot more pleasure in it."

Bottom line: If you judge yourself, you'll feel bad, which triggers old circuits of emotional eating—eating to make yourself feel better. But if you're gentle with yourself to start with—and mindfulness cultivates gentleness—you'll create new brain circuits around eating.

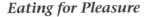

Eating for Pleasure

My colleague Jon Kabat-Zinn, Ph.D., who founded the Center for Mindfulness in Medicine, Health Care, and Society, invented a mindful-eating exercise that you might enjoy. After all, if you're eating that pie, why waste it by wolfing it down in a few bites while you're thinking about something else? Isn't that how a lot of eating happens? How about concentrating on what you're eating and extracting every last bit of pleasure out of it?

Kabat-Zinn Raisin Exercise

1. **Examine a single raisin carefully for a minute or so.** Observe the end where the stem was, the wrinkles, the shape, the texture . . . whatever you can notice. When you and the raisin are on intimate terms, then pop it into your mouth. No chewing yet!

2. **Roll the raisin around on your tongue**, exploring its curves and wrinkles. Yes, of course, eating is sensuous.

3. **Puncture the raisin with your teeth**, and notice what happens. Are you salivating? Is your throat opening? What's the burst of flavor like? What else is happening?

4. **Chew the raisin slowly**, observing all the sensations.

5. **Swallow the raisin**, and notice how interesting and complex the process is.

If you try this exercise even once, it will make eating a much more enjoyable experience. It also slows the process down. If you find yourself eating fast, put your fork down, take a breath, and resume at a slower, more mindful pace. Eating slowly gives the brain time to register fullness, and you'll naturally eat less.

You can do anything mindfully, and when you do, life becomes a lot more fun and interesting. If you take a mindful shower, you'll enjoy the sensation of water and heat, suds and massage. That beats spending your shower time reviewing your anxieties or pitching a fit over that belly fat. If you're making love, make love instead of mentally composing your grocery list. When you choose a couple of activities to do mindfully every day, you'll be changing your brain *and* your attitude.

Fun, pleasure, and creativity evolve naturally out of the brain hygiene that mindfulness trains. And, of course, you'll slowly gain the advantage over cravings. But when a craving wins, at least you'll enjoy it without falling into a cycle of emotional eating.

Breakfast Eating and Mindfulness

An Israeli research team, led by Professor Daniela Jakubowicz of Tel Aviv University's Sackler Faculty of Medicine, gives a thumbs-up to eating a big breakfast.[1] *Science Daily* summarized her research: "In a study of nearly 200 clinically obese, nondiabetic adults, a researcher found that a 600-calorie breakfast that includes dessert as well as proteins and carbohydrates can help dieters lose weight and keep it off over the long term. Her research indicates that such a morning meal staves off cravings and defuses psychological addictions to sweet foods."

Were you paying attention? A big breakfast that *includes* dessert helps people lose weight? Let me explain.

The study compared two groups of obese and overweight people who were allowed the same number of calories each day. One group ate a big breakfast that included a dessert. (Yes, that did infuriate almost all nutritionists.) The other experimental group ate a small breakfast so that more calories were left for lunch and dinner. At the end of 16 weeks, both groups had lost the same amount of weight. But in a follow-up period, the small-breakfast group gained back an average of 24 pounds (75 percent of what they'd lost), while the big-breakfast group lost an average of 15 more pounds. That's a huge difference, literally and figuratively.

Professor Jakubowicz attributes the success of the breakfast splurgers to fewer cravings and a reduction in *ghrelin,* the hunger hormone. In another study, she showed that the metabolic indicators of the big-breakfast eaters improved as well. The group that ate a small breakfast, in contrast, felt more deprived, which led them to cheat on their diets over time and gain the weight back.

But here's an interesting question, posed in an article in the *New York Times* by journalist Anahad O'Connor: Did the big-breakfast group profit because of a physiological effect on cravings, or was it a psychological effect? After all, eating a big breakfast with dessert is a stunning departure from the usual dietary advice. It's an oddball behavior. So let's take a look at an earlier study that O'Connor reviewed, published in the *American Journal of Clinical Nutrition*. It was carried out way back in 1992, by researchers from the department of psychology at Vanderbilt University. The study adds a surprising twist to the breakfast question.[2]

When moderately obese people who habitually skipped breakfast were asked to eat it while on a calorie-controlled diet, they lost an average of 17 pounds in 12 weeks. Okay, that seems to substantiate the Jakubowicz study. But when another group who usually ate breakfast were put on the same diet and asked to skip breakfast, they lost an average of almost 20 pounds. The difference between the two groups was not significant.[3]

If both the breakfast eaters and the breakfast skippers essentially lost the same amount of weight, where does that leave us? According to O'Connor, both programs included an "identical amount of calories, and each caused people to lose more weight than a program in which a person's typical breakfast habits did not change. The study was fairly small and limited, involving only 52 overweight adult women, but *it suggested that as far as breakfast is concerned, the most important factor in weight loss may be how drastically you change your routine* [emphasis mine]."[4]

Chalk up another point for mindfulness. Changing your routine diverts thought and behavior off the familiar beaten path. Old brain circuits that governed your previous eating behaviors slowly stop firing. New brain circuits then form, and the rewiring slowly transforms your behavior. This happens under the table, so to speak (in an unconscious way), so that willpower isn't involved.

The brain, through its inherent genius for neuroplasticity, changes itself, and you reap the benefits.

So what's the bottom line? Is it better to eat breakfast or not? As researchers are always saying, more research is needed. In the meantime, you are your own best lab rat.

See what happens if you eat a big breakfast for a few days or a week. For dessert, have one of my surprisingly delicious low-carb almond flour cookies (naturally gluten-free) or a piece of almond-flour bread with a small amount of jam—just a teaspoon of fruit spread to avoid blood-sugar spikes. Alternatively, you may choose to experiment with skipping breakfast for a while if you habitually eat it. The choice is yours.

The bread and cookie recipes for your experiment are in Part IV of the book. And believe me, PlantPlus baked treats are the best! Rich in protein and good fats, they're very satisfying. You won't feel deprived when you eat these.

By the way, the old advice to eat breakfast because it promotes better health was based on flawed observational studies that can't prove causation. One more science myth bites the dust. So unless you're pregnant or have an illness that requires eating frequent meals, don't worry that skipping breakfast might harm your health. In fact, there's evidence that intermittent fasting (say, after dinner to lunch) may increase longevity. And since fasting means that you're not releasing insulin—the fat-storing hormone—it can also lead to weight loss. What a deal.

In this chapter, we've covered how to fight cravings and retrain your brain through mindfulness and self-awareness. If you do the breathing exercise a few times a day (whenever you feel stuck or when a craving strikes), you'll be laying down new neural pathways. Likewise, try to incorporate some mindfulness exercises in your day. Water the plants mindfully—enjoying the sights and smells instead of wishing you were done. Eat a piece of dark chocolate with complete dedication to the experience. Stroke the dog or cat with full attention. Listen to your kids, spouse, or coworker without thinking about something else. An alternate word for this mindful approach to life is *love*.

Another way to create mindfulness and form new brain circuits is to clean out your kitchen. Those stale crackers, frozen bagels, candy bars, and such need to find a new home. When you clean out the old, you make room for the new. And the new look of your kitchen, cabinets, and the contents of the refrigerator and the pantry will create more mindfulness in you and make way for the PlantPlus reformation.

Out with habit and in with awareness! That's the subject of our next chapter.

CHAPTER 22

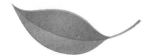

Your Sleek, New PlantPlus Kitchen:

Out with the Old and "Inn" with the New

*"If you want something new, you have
to stop doing something old."*

— Peter F. Drucker

Inn with the new? Did the editors fail to catch a misprint? Not at all. When you carry out the recommendations in this chapter, your kitchen will feel more like an inn than a place to do chores. You'll be both innkeeper and guest, all set up to live happily in your own PlantPlus heaven. This is the last Lifestyle Bite, the final preparation before you actually start your new way of life with the Reboot in Part III.

Cleaning out the old is a mindful activity that restores attention and awareness. For example, sometimes I clean out the pantry because I've spotted (pardon me, if you're eating) mouse poop. These little critters abound in our mountain habitat, and if I forget to put edibles into mouse-proof containers, they mosey right in for a snack. It always amazes me what's hiding in the pantry. Lost bottles of olive oil. Mouse-chewed napkins. Old tea bags that someone sent for Christmas three years ago. Empty bottles of spice. Clam juice that has been aging in the bottle for 20 years like fine wine.

When Gordon and I clean off the shelves, toss out the old stuff, and reorganize, we always feel a sense of lightness and accomplishment. We know what's in there, what's not in there, and what we need to buy. Sometimes the things we discover even give us inspiration for making a new dish or two. But what's always amazing to us both is that the very act of cleaning out the old leaves us feeling renewed. That makes cleaning a ritual act.

What's the Heck's a Ritual?

A *ritual* is anything with transformative potential. On the Jewish celebration of Passover, for example, the central ritual involves giving up leavened wheat products, although that's certainly not how my ancestors would have framed it!

During the eight days of Passover, it's forbidden to eat anything leavened, in memory of the Exodus from Egypt, which happened so fast that there wasn't time to let the bread rise. Unleavened bread (matzah) could be baked in the sun on top of a wagon as the Jews fled, so it's the only gluten-containing food that our tribe is allowed to consume during the eight-day Passover celebration.

In preparation for Passover, observant Jews take everything out of their cupboards. Some people even sweep the shelves with a feather. The point is to chase out even the tiniest crumb of leaven and then—in a beautiful ceremony—cast it into running water.

Sweeping out the leaven isn't just about food, of course. It's a metaphor for sweeping out all the things that hold us hostage: stress, a life that's too complex, bad relationships, and limiting beliefs and outmoded behaviors that no longer serve us. Passover is a celebration of the freedom to become our authentic selves, and in the process help others become free from oppression and enslavement—both internal and external.

Eating the PlantPlus way is also a celebration of freedom from some of life's unnecessary complexity. Streamlining your kitchen and your food choices, trimming down prep time for meals, saving money, and eliminating the need to eat health-destroying fast food gives you more degrees of freedom than you may have thought possible.

During Passover, special plates and cooking utensils are used for the duration of the eight-day holiday. Changing up your pots, pans, and dishes is a powerful cue for the brain and mind. It's a symbolic act, a declaration of change.

Research shows that one small change—like using small plates instead of dinner plates—can help you lose weight independent of any other variables. The smaller the plate, the less food gets piled on it as well. And if you eat slowly and mindfully, enjoying every bite, you're likely to feel sated before you've eaten excessively.

Changing up your plates is just the beginning of streamlining your kitchen for a more conscious food lifestyle.

The Big, Fat Kitchen Cleanse

One year after a sadly contentious divorce, I comforted myself by watching late-night cookware infomercials. You don't have to be Freud to figure out that nurture was on my mind. After all, that's what eating is all about. I stepped up to the plate with a check for 400 hard-earned bucks (a measure of my desperation) for what turned out to be a flimsy set of nonstick cookware. It bit the dust within the year, leaving a trail of nasty chemicals in its wake.

Did I really think that a nonstick surface could be good for me? Especially when it started to scratch and slowly flake off? I guess I was too busy to think about it. Over the years since that time, a lot more pots and pans have come and gone.

Let's take a quick look at how to create your sleek PlantPlus kitchen. Use your imagination and creativity, as long as you bring in items that are useful, healthful, and inspiring. My advice to you is this: Be merciless, and stand your ground. If you don't love the stuff in your kitchen, give it to somebody else. You're turning over a whole new leaf, and your kitchen cleanse is a symbol of that with the power to change your mind and your brain.

Out with the Old:
Pots, Pans, Dishes, Utensils,
Appliances, and Knickknacks

- **Nonstick cookware**: Don't kid yourself. You're eating toxic chemicals when you use this kind of cookware. Don't give it away. Recycle it.

- **Plastic items** like ladles, stirring spoons, spatulas, storage containers, cutting boards, mugs and glasses, baby plates, spoons, bottles, and thermal mugs. If you microwave foods (this is a controversial subject that we don't need to get into here), use glass or ceramic. Never heat any food in a plastic container or plastic wrap.

- **Dishes, cups, and glasses:** Think about what you like to eat and drink from. Is it aesthetically pleasing? Eating should be a pleasure rather than a trip to the dump. Look around at what has outlived its usefulness. What about that old Cookie Monster mug or the hideous serving dish that Aunt Emily gave you when you married your ex-husband? What about the cheesy dishes you brought home from Goodwill years ago and never use? What a relief it will be to bring them all to the thrift shop.

- **Old appliances**: Our kitchen counter was crowded with various gadgets for slicing and dicing, blending and pureeing, toasting, roasting, mixing, and coffee making. Unless an appliance was in use daily, or near daily, we either moved it to the bottom shelf of our pantry out of sight or gave it away. If you're not sure that you're ready to give up that ancient electric breadmaker, put it into storage. Otherwise, bring used appliances to the thrift store. Clutter saps energy and uses up valuable counter space that you'll be needing to whip up all those delicious PlantPlus meals.

- **Odds and ends:** When my mom died, I took some of her old baking pans. They had a lot of memories in them. After 25 years, they'd gotten older still. I kept a couple as heirlooms, but I finally recycled the old browned and dented cookie sheets, knives too old and dull to work with, warped baking tins, and rusted sugar-cookie cutters. We brought at least ten glass vases, left from flowers we'd been given over the years, to Goodwill as well. What have you got to recycle? How about those souvenir Eiffel Tower salt-and-pepper shakers and knickknacks of all kinds that have outlived their cuteness and joined the world of kitsch?

Inn with the New

One way to become a better cook is to have the right pots, pans, and tools. Most of the equipment you need is simple, inexpensive, and long lasting, like my favorite cast-iron frying pan. The few items that are pricey—enamel pots and pans, and perhaps a Vitamix blender—can often be bought used or on sale. This is a list of a few of my favorite things, many of them specialized for PlantPlus cooking. You, of course, will make your own list.

- **Dutch oven:** Our earthy-red Le Creuset Dutch oven is our prized cooking pot. Yes, it's heavy—a wonderful addition to any fitness program. Ours is frequently in use, simmering a fragrant soup or stew. Because these pots are made of cast iron, they conduct heat evenly so that food is much less likely to burn. The enamel surface is nonreactive so that nothing nasty leaches into your food. Furthermore, the pot goes from the stove right into the fridge when the contents are cool enough, serving as a storage container. We scoop out enough for a meal and leave the rest for another day. Marshalls, Costco, and other discount chains often have high-quality enamel cookware at reasonable prices. They're worth the money because they last for years. In fact, they might just become family heirlooms.

- **Slow cooker:** If I'm home to stir a pot, I often make one-dish meals in the Dutch oven. If I'm going out, I use a slow cooker. Put the ingredients in before you leave the house, and return to the fragrance of a perfectly cooked meal. I might whip up some coq au vin in there or perhaps a tasty vegetable soup.

- **Cast-iron and/or enamel frying pans:** Gordon uses our Le Creuset enamel-clad cast-iron omelet pan several times a week, both for omelets and for sautéing vegetables. We also have a 15-inch cast-iron frying pan that I bought at Marshalls for about $15. Instead of deteriorating over time, cast-iron pans improve with age once they are oiled and heated so that the surface becomes nonstick. You can find instructions on the Web for how to season cast iron. Here's a simple rule of thumb: If your food sticks, it's not seasoned correctly. A properly seasoned cast-iron pan has the best nonstick surface of them all.

- **Cutting boards:** You'll be chopping a lot of veggies, so a couple of good cutting boards (one just for meat, if you eat it) are a necessity. Silicone cutting boards can release bits of fiberglass into your food, so they're out. Glass boards are noisy and unpleasant, and they dull your knives fast. Plastic can leach hormone disruptors into your food. Wood, on the other hand, is harder to clean. You can read everything you'd ever want to know about cutting boards in one article at www.kitchenstewardship.com/2012/09/17/monday -mission-examine-your-cutting-board. The author cites a source stating that "in a UC Davis study comparing scratched-up wooden and plastic cutting boards, the wooden boards were found to be naturally antimicrobial, while plastic cutting boards allowed more bacteria to thrive, even after being washed." Live and learn. I put our wooden boards in the dishwasher to disinfect from time to time, and then rub them back to life with olive oil.

- **Blender:** After our old blender gave out, we saved our pennies and sprang for a Vitamix because it can blend absolutely anything. The Vitamix is great for making smoothies without the need to peel ingredients like ginger or turmeric root. You don't even need to core apples. Just cut them into chunks and toss them in, seeds and all. Whereas juicing removes the valuable fiber from fruits and veggies, blending them gives you whole-foods nutrition. You can sometimes get a used Vitamix on Craigslist, but for most uses, an inexpensive blender with a glass container works well enough. Check the reviews on Amazon to be assured of getting one with a strong motor.

- **Set of stainless pots:** We have a basic set of good stainless-steel pots (small, medium, and large with a handy steamer insert) to boil eggs, steam vegetables, make sauces, and the like. These are priced reasonably at discount stores and provide a nonreactive, food-safe cooking surface.

- **Mini food processor.** We got ours for $25 at Macy's. This little gem is handy for chopping onions and garlic, creating sauces, and what have you.

- **Small coffee grinder.** One-cup coffee grinders (as cheap as $10 on Amazon) are wonderful for grinding fresh spices.

- **Salad spinner:** Yup, these are plastic, but you've got to pick your battles. Look for a BPA-free model. What better way to wash your greens and herbs? It's fun for the kids, too.

- **Set of glass measuring cups:** A three-piece set (one-cup, two-cup, and four-cup) should cover most of your needs.

- **Two sets of stainless measuring cups:** These sets usually contain a quarter-, third-, half-, and one-cup measures. These are essential for baking, and the extra set comes in handy when the other one is dirty.

- **Two sets of stainless measuring spoons:** These sets usually contain a quarter-teaspoon, half-teaspoon, one-teaspoon, and one-tablespoon measures. Ditto the need for two sets.

- **Glass storage containers:** Use glass containers (most have plastic tops) for storing everything from nuts, to nut flours, to leftovers. You can get them at discount stores for a reasonable price.

- **Baking sheets:** A heavy-duty stainless baking sheet with sides for roasting vegetables, and two stainless-steel cookie sheets, should do the job.

- **Cooling racks:** Two metal racks for cooling bread, crackers, and cookies.

- **Stainless-steel and wood kitchen utensils:** This includes spatulas, ladles, and stirring spoons. When the plastic went out, these babies came in.

- **Hand mixer:** We rarely use this electric gadget, but every once in a while, it still comes in handy for things like whipping cream or making meringue.

- **Glass jars:** Mason jars work well for fermenting veggies or making pickles on your very own countertop. It's also wise to save some of the glass jars that foods come packed in. These are perfect for storage and for sharing your bounty with friends, since presumably they won't have to worry about giving your old glass bottles back unless you've become attached to them. In that case, I can recommend a good therapist.

- **Misto:** A Misto is a refillable sprayer. Sleek little things made of stainless steel, they have a built-in pump that you activate with a few pushes on the top. We keep ours filled with olive oil to spray in the frying pan or on veggies before roasting. You could put avocado oil in a Misto when you want a more neutral oil for greasing baking dishes or cookie sheets. Costco sometimes has two-packs of Mistos cheap.

- **Baking pan: 3½" x 7".** This is the size in which we bake our delicious loaves of almond bread. If you've got a mind to do that, get one of these pans first.

- **Use your imagination**, but keep in mind that less is more. Clutter not only wastes money but also makes the kitchen feel less spacious and pleasant.

Once again, I implore you: Be merciless in your cleaning out, and choose carefully what you bring in. Even if your budget doesn't allow for a complete kitchen makeover, you can purchase one or two items that will make a big difference. The one item that I use daily and that waits always ready on the stovetop is our big cast-iron frying pan. Though inexpensive, it's especially precious. That one $15 pan symbolizes the entire transformation to PlantPlus for us. It's our mindful reminder that we're on a delicious journey that makes our lives healthier, happier, and a lot more fun.

🍃 🍃 🍃

Now it's time to move on to Part III, and there are only two chapters in this section. The first teaches you the PlantPlus Reboot, and the second chapter is all about how to personalize your PlantPlus lifestyle. Read through these, and whadya know? Pretty soon, you'll get to Part IV: Let's Eat!

PART III

GETTING DOWN TO BUSINESS

I hope you're excited about trading in your old lifestyle for a new, healthier one. But even though you're ready to start, you may also be a little bit anxious. *Will I like real food? Will I miss processed food? Will my kids adapt or pitch a fit?*

Some people are bound to adjust more easily to a PlantPlus lifestyle than others. But no worries—even picky kids will come around when parents set a good example. You can do it. I know you can! I believe in you. So in this short, practical section, I'll make things as simple as I can to set you up for your new lifestyle launch.

When a friend of mine decided to give PlantPlus a try, she was scared because she didn't know where to start. She looked at me with big eyes, threw her hands up in the air, and pleaded, "Make me a list. Be specific. I need to know what to get rid of and what to stock up on. I'm a beginner here, so cut me a break." I did, and you're the beneficiary of this step-by-step approach to falling in love with real food.

The first step in your food makeover is what I call the Reboot, a four-week program of healthy, carb-reasonable eating. Is it a cleanse? That's a popular word right now. Well, yes, of course, it's a *cleanse* when you dump processed foods and extra carbs, but there's no need to fast or forego all your pleasures. You'll just discover new pleasures.

The second step in your food makeover is personalizing your PlantPlus lifestyle. This process is also simple. Personalization is an ongoing process because we're always changing. Our age, stress level, and even where we live affects our metabolism. In this chapter, you'll read the stories of several of my colleagues who made the conversion to PlantPlus and what it has been like for them to completely change up the way they eat. Inspiring!

What you'll be learning is how to be mindful, aware, and flexible —and to personalize your nutrition for life.

CHAPTER 23

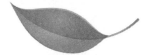

Reboot:

What's On and Off the Menu

"If it comes from a plant, <u>eat it.</u>
If it's made in a plant, <u>don't.</u>"

— Mee Tracy McCormick

Here's the vision: Within a month of rebooting your diet, you'll be well on your way to becoming a whole new person—quite literally:

> "Your body is constantly replacing old cells with new ones at the rate of millions per second. By the time you finish reading this sentence, 50 million of your cells will have died and been replaced by others."[1]

So just how much of your body *can* you replace?

Larry Dossey, M.D.—one of the great science commentators of our time—cites data from radio-isotope studies indicating that approximately 98 percent of the 10^{28} atoms in our bodies are replaced every year. At a more macro level, the cells lining your stomach are renewed weekly. The cells lining the surface of your small intestine and colon are renewed every four to six days. Bone turns over quickly, too. Osteoclasts remove old bone, while osteoblasts lay down new bone with such dedication that roughly 10 percent of your skeleton is replaced every year. All cells and tissues have their own rates of turnover and renewal—a continual cycle of death and rebirth that goes on until you die.[2]

But what about the remaining 90 percent of your cells—the tiny microbial beasties with whom you cohabit and coevolve? Bacteria divide approximately every 20 minutes. So let's say you have one bacterium of a certain species in your gut at 9:00 A.M. It divides into two at about 9:20 A.M. The two daughter cells each divide at about 9:40, and now there are four identical bacteria. The four divide into eight, and so on down the line in a rapidly expanding logarithmic progression. By 4 P.M., there are already 2,000,000 cells.

> Within days, and even hours, of a dietary change, the composition and number of bacteria in your gut ecosystem also changes, as does their gene expression.[3] That makes sense in terms of ancestral hunter-gatherer cultures that had to adapt to a constantly changing food supply.

Here's the bottom line: It's never too late to renew your body by changing your diet. Whether you're young or old, your body is more resilient than you might think. So are you ready? Let's get started on your atomic, molecular, structural, metabolic, immune, and mood makeover.

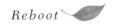

The PlantPlus Reboot

For four weeks, you'll be eliminating some foods from your diet and adding others as outlined in this section. It may or may not be easy to change your diet at first. It's human nature to take comfort in the familiar and be suspicious of the new. But it's also easy to form new habits if you have the information, inspiration, and intention to improve your life and that of your family's.

The four-week Reboot doesn't last forever, and the foods are very tasty. Bear in mind that some of the foods you eliminated in the Reboot can be added back later when you personalize the diet for your metabolism, although you may opt to stick with the Reboot foods because they're delicious and make you feel great. That's been true for me. I eat pretty much the same foods after two years that I did for the first four weeks. The only difference is that I let myself have an occasional off-plan meal when we're out on the town or at the home of friends.

The process of adapting to a new diet can feel like moving to a new house. At first you might be a little anxious, convinced that you'll miss the familiarity of your old home. But as soon as you move, there's a lot to do. It's fun to settle in and create a new way of life. Commitment to rebooting any aspect of life gives you energy—and the energy feels like fun. Mastering something new is an exciting, empowering experience.

What's Off the Menu

- **Grain:** This includes whole grains, pseudograins like quinoa, and grain flour. Common examples are wheat, corn, barley, oats, amaranth, rice, bulgur, spelt, faro, millet, buckwheat, rye, sorghum, teff, triticale, and wild rice. It doesn't matter if the grain in question has gluten or not. All whole grains and all flours are off the table for the Reboot.

- **Sugar**: This includes obvious sources of sugar like honey, agave, maple syrup, brown sugar, white sugar, raw sugar, coconut sugar, barley syrup, cane juice, molasses, brown-rice syrup, and so on. Even organic dehydrated cane juice, which sounds so healthful (and goes by the name *rapadura*) is just another word for sugar. Some natural foods, such as dried fruits and all fruit juices, are also high in sugar and not appropriate for the Reboot. Artificial sweeteners are also off the menu. You can use the natural sweetener stevia if you'd like.

- **Processed foods**: Almost all processed foods are high in sugar, fat, and salt—or in the case of the ubiquitous low-fat processed foods, high in sugar and salt. Many are also made with GMO ingredients and laced with chemicals and preservatives.

- **High-starch vegetables,** including white potatoes, sweet potatoes, yams, peas, winter squash, plantains, yucca, and water chestnuts.

- **Legumes,** primarily beans and peanuts.

- **"Industrial" vegetable oils**: These include cottonseed, sunflower, safflower, corn, canola, and grapeseed oil; blended vegetable oils; commercial heat-extracted olive oil; margarine; and solid shortening.

- **Beer**: The hops that most beers are brewed from contain gluten. Even gluten-free beers are brewed from grain, may contain an excessive amount of carbohydrates, and can defeat the purpose of your diet experiment. Read more about this in the beer and wine list to come.

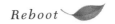
What's On the Menu (for Omnivores)

- **Vegetables:** One pound of low-starch vegetables a day (see Chapter 27 to understand what this looks like) in as large a variety and as many colors as you can round up.

- **Fruit:** If your weight is good, two or three pieces of whole fruit a day. One cup of berries is the equivalent of one fruit. Limit high-sugar fruits like banana, pineapple, mango, and papaya to half-cup servings once in a while (twice a week or less). If you're overweight or have metabolic problems, limit your daily fruit to a half cup of berries—the lowest-sugar fruit—until you reach your target weight.

- **Protein:** Wild-caught, sustainable fish; pasture-raised poultry, meat, and whole eggs.

- **Nuts and seeds:** Nuts and seeds are high in phytonutrients, good fats, and good fiber, as well as containing some protein. They're filling, incredibly handy, and taste great.

- **Fermented foods** that have live probiotics like yogurt, kefir, sauerkraut, kimchi, and pickles, as long as they haven't been heated to kill the precious probiotic bacteria.

- **Organic dairy from pastured cows,** unless you're lactose intolerant, have an allergy to milk protein, or are vegan.

- **Healthy oils** that are organic, nonGMO, and cold pressed: extra-virgin olive oil, sesame oil (for salads, not sautéing), avocado oil, and coconut oil.

- **Healthy animal fats:** Ghee (melted butter without the solids), butter, and fat from wild-caught fish and pasture-raised poultry and meat.

- **Tea and coffee** unless you're anxious or have a mood disorder. Water-processed (not chemically processed) decaffeinated tea or coffee is okay if caffeine doesn't work for you.

- **Chocolate**: Two tablespoons of fair-trade, unsweetened, organic cocoa powder a day, or two squares of organic dark chocolate (minimum 55 percent cacao).

Vegan and Vegetarian Menu Amendments

Because your protein sources are limited, you'll need to make a few changes in the Reboot menu. Try amending your Reboot list to include starchy vegetables, such as sweet potatoes and other tubers. Add legumes as long as you first soak them for 8 to 12 hours to reduce tannins, phytates, and other antinutrients.

Soy is a controversial protein source, but remember that it's a staple of the Japanese, a very long-lived people. The reason for the soy controversy is threefold: First, soybeans (like all legumes) are rich in antinutrient phytates. These inhibit your gut from absorbing certain minerals like calcium, magnesium, iron, and zinc. Second, soybeans are a big GMO crop. Third, soy is a common cause of adverse food reactions.

One of my friends and colleagues, Marilyn Tam—former CEO of Aveda; former president of Reebok Apparel and Retail Group; and a successful entrepreneur, speaker, and author of *The Happiness Choice* and *How to Use What You've Got to Get What You Want*—has considerable expertise in nutrition. She has a degree in foods and nutrition from Oregon State University and co-owned and operated an integrated health clinic for several years.

At the clinic, they found that integrating leading-edge science with the wisdom of traditional medicine, which places a large emphasis on nutrition and listening to one's body, led to the most improvement in physical, mental, and emotional health—and provided the most lasting results. Marilyn is a long-term (more than

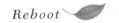

20 years), mostly grain-free vegan whose protein comes largely from vegetables, nuts, beans, lentils, and tempeh—the healthiest form of soy since it's fermented and low in antinutrients.

Marilyn is always open to changing her diet based on what she learns and observes about her own health. That kind of curious attitude prevents what humorist Loretta LaRoche calls "hardening of the attitude." Marilyn agreed to be interviewed, and I'd like to share an excerpt of our conversation:

> *Joan*: Marilyn, you're the most disciplined eater that I've ever met.
>
> *Marilyn*: I don't think of it as discipline; it's just how I am. To eat something outside of what I know is good for me feels shocking. Why would I eat sugar? It's not a food group. I don't eat things that aren't food. I also like to eat lower on the food chain. I don't make any judgments—I just think that this way of eating is good for me as part of the food chain. I'm part of the cycle of life, and we're all entitled to live. I can have less impact on the Earth by not eating meat. But if someone eats meat because that's what they need to sustain themselves, I have no judgment.

Marilyn's diet changes with the season and with what's fresh and available. In the winter, for example, she eats less salad and more root vegetables, beans, peas, and lentils. When I had the good fortune of being her guest for dinner one evening, she roasted beets, kabocha squash, fennel, onion, parsnips, and tempeh. The process was amazingly simple. Marilyn melted a small scoop of coconut oil in a big, flat baking pan, added a variety of seasonings, and then added the vegetables, stirred to coat them, and baked them for 40 minutes or so. Look for some of Marilyn's recipes, including her Power Smoothie, in Chapter 27. Whether you're a vegan, a vegetarian, or an omnivore, you'll enjoy her tasty, healthful culinary treats.

What about Wine, Beer, and Spirits?

I love a glass of good red wine, so the question about whether to drink alcohol or not is close to my heart—and to my breasts, as well. There's literature suggesting that alcohol leads to an increase in the incidence of breast cancer. A lot of the studies, however, are the observational type that can establish association, but can't prove causation. Abstinence from alcohol, for example, might be a proxy for healthful eating, exercise, or other protective health habits.

Not knowing what to think, I consulted the website of my old friend, breast-cancer surgeon Susan Love, M.D. She quoted a meta-analysis (a study of studies) of the observational data linking alcohol consumption to breast cancer. Women who drank alcohol had a 22 percent increase in the *relative* risk (this, as you'll see, is not the same as *absolute* risk) of developing breast cancer. Dr. Love pointed out that for every additional daily drink, there was a 10 percent increase in relative risk, meaning that if your risk is 10 percent, it will increase to 11 percent. Fortunately, she asserts, good eating habits can offset whatever small risk there might be:

> Several large studies show [that] high intake of folic acid, found in spinach, broccoli, corn, legumes, and multivitamins, appeared to mitigate the excess risk of breast cancer from alcohol. Since one to two drinks a day have been shown to decrease heart disease, this gives those of you who enjoy your cocktail or glass of wine an out: increase your green leafy vegetables and take a multivitamin.[4]

Dr. Love concludes her analysis by asking the big question that nutritional research in general poses: How can we make up our minds about whether to drink alcohol or not when there isn't really enough good information?

"The breast-cancer risk increase isn't great," she writes, "but it definitely exists. You alone know how much pleasure you get from your glass of wine or beer, and how alarmed you are at the thought of breast cancer."[5]

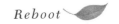

So, dear reader, make your own decision about whether or not to drink alcohol. The National Institutes of Health defines a "standard drink" as:

- 5 ounces of wine (there are approximately five drinks in a standard 750 ml bottle)

- 12 ounces of regular beer

- 1.5 ounces of distilled spirits

If you do decide to drink alcohol, don't add any sugary stuff to your spirits. Avoid simple syrup (sugar water); drink mixes (sugar and chemicals); and cordials like Triple Sec and Grand Marnier used as mixers (11 grams of carbs and 100 calories in a single ounce).

So is light beer a good choice for after the Reboot? Maybe or maybe not. Most light beers are brewed from hops and contain gluten. So here's an experiment that a beer drinker might do: Google gluten-free light beer after the Reboot, and you'll come up with several brands. Give one a try, and see how it works taste-wise and gut-wise for you.

What to Expect on the Reboot

A Reboot heads-up: You might feel worse briefly before you start to feel better. Or you may just feel better straightaway.

The *low-carb flu*, which generally resolves quickly, is sometimes reported when people cut back on the amount of carbs they consume. The symptoms can include fatigue, light-headedness, foggy brain, achiness, irritability, anxiety, and sleep disturbances. These adjustment-related symptoms usually disappear within a week or two at most.

Gordon didn't experience any adjustment symptoms, but I did. I became dizzy and light-headed. After a few days of that, however, instead of the fatigue that some people report, I experienced a burst of energy. But it was hard to concentrate and difficult to sleep, and I thought that the diet just wasn't for me. I wrote as much on my Facebook page, reporting on:

> The food experiment . . . I've lost two pounds so far; had megatrouble sleeping, which is rare for me; significant problems with digestion; light-headedness; and irritability. I'm also flying high! The food is very satisfying, so there is no hunger—just a growing feeling that this diet does not suit my body type. I'll try it for another week and report back.

Fortunately, all the adjustment symptoms were gone by the end of the first week, and I was feeling better than I had in years.

What about weight? It's typical for a woman to lose three to five pounds during the first week of any low-carb diet. Men often lose more. Most of the weight loss will be water and feces, but a pound or two will be fat. Losing one or two pounds a week thereafter is a reasonable expectation. It's also advisable not to lose the weight any more quickly, since the slower the weight loss, the less loose skin you're likely to end up with.

Josh, a friend and colleague who works in the field of Chinese medicine and nutrition, lost 55 pounds over 7 months—and 75 pounds after 18 months—when he decided to try a PlantPlus Diet experiment. His life partner, Keith, an acupuncturist, lost 25 pounds during that same time. You'll read more about their experiences later.

I want to emphasize that **if you notice physical changes in symptoms that might have required medication—or may suddenly require medication—it's imperative to discuss them with your physician rather than changing medications on your own.**

CHAPTER 24

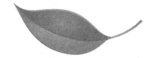

Personalization:

Your Own
PlantPlus Lifestyle

*"There's no way you can fail 'the diet';
you can only discover your own."*

— Angela Thomas, R.N.

Most popular books on diet and nutrition feature case histories of people who were overweight and had health problems but who are now lean and thriving. That's what piques our interest. He lost 333 pounds? (That's an actual case in Dr. Joel Fuhrman's best-selling book *Eat to Live*.) She lost 30 pounds? (That's a case in Jorge Cruise's *Belly Fat Cure*.) These cases are great because they mobilize our excitement and resolve. If he can do it, or if she can do it, then so can I!

So I thought I'd include a few case studies for you. What makes them so interesting is that each person's experience led him or her to eat foods that were quite different, although all the participants eat plant-rich diets. Since I'm not a diet doctor or a health coach, I don't have clients. But as a scientist and psychologist, I do have colleagues who are health professionals. Several of them volunteered to try the PlantPlus way of eating and share their experiences.

Angela Thomas, a holistic nurse, lost 15 pounds in eight months, reversed her prediabetes, and lowered her inflammation. My friend and noted acupuncturist Keith lost 25 pounds, and his partner, Josh, lost 75 pounds. I also interviewed several other colleagues who had previously developed their own whole-foods, personalized diets based on a foundation of plants.

Each of these colleagues agreed to be interviewed in order to share their experiences and insights with you. In this chapter, you'll read some of their stories, and then I'll coach you on how to personalize your own diet. Let's start with my good friend Angela, a holistic nurse and nurse coach.

Angela

> *Joan*: What made you want to try a PlantPlus Diet experiment?

> *Angela*: It was my health. I had an autoimmune condition, asthma, prediabetes, belly fat, and carb cravings. I knew as a nurse that the belly fat was a cytokine factory that was related to my high levels of inflammation. I was also fatigued a lot and suspected that my diet was a factor. At conferences, I noticed that after eating carbs, I'd want to sleep through the afternoon lecture. But if I ate a salad and lean protein, I didn't have that dip in energy. I used to make brown rice every week and eat it daily—part of a healthy macrobiotic diet—but I just couldn't lose any weight.

Angela lost five pounds in the first few weeks of her PlantPlus Reboot. At first, following the diet was difficult. Angela felt light-headed and had to watch out for low blood sugar, but after the first few weeks, she was feeling much better. Her inflammatory markers were down, her energy was improved, and a rash on her face related to her autoimmune condition completely disappeared.

After several weeks, she decided to test her response to gluten-free baked goods, which she now calls "a red flag for anyone who wants to be healthy." The gluten-free products stalled her weight loss, so she stopped eating grains for the most part, except for the occasional meal out. Over the next six months, she lost a total of 15 pounds.

Angela's advice is this:

> You need to pay attention to how you feel. There are a zillion diets out there, and new information comes out every day, so treat your diet like an experiment. Let go of ideas about what's right and what's wrong, and just be curious. See what happens. Be mindful.
>
> When I tell people that I feel better on this diet, there are always naysayers who tell me I'm wrong. "You took brown rice out? That's ridiculous! It's so healthy." Don't listen to what other people say; rather, know what is true for you. It comes down to honoring your own experience.
>
> We all have to find our comfort foods that are healthy, and to live like this, you need to plan. You can't get almond bread at the corner deli, for instance. When you challenge yourself with foods that make you feel bad, though, that's powerful motivation to get back on track.

Mee

Mee Tracy McCormick, author of *My Kitchen Cure*, which became an almost instantaneous sensation when she self-published it in 2013, began to explore her diet out of necessity. When I first met Mee (short for Meghan), she was like a bone—so thin that a wind might pick her up and carry her away.

Mee had endured years of crippling intestinal pain. Her major memory of young adulthood—and every vacation she ever went on—always involved debilitating pain. Her digestive tract was ulcerated, and she couldn't absorb enough nutrients to sustain herself.

Mee's mother died of Crohn's disease, and Mee was headed in the same direction. However, today—four years after becoming a diet sleuth—Mee is healthy and pain-free. She's also an accomplished chef and TV personality.

Her fabulously informative down-home book is called *My Kitchen Cure* for a reason. She knows that it may not be *Your* Kitchen Cure because the feedback from each of our bodies is what guides us in the healing journey. The process of finding her own way back to health empowered Mee, and it will empower you, too.

Mee wants you to know the following:

> When you go into the kitchen and find your own cure, you learn how capable you really are. I once thought I wasn't capable, wasn't talented enough. I'm not Dr. Oz, after all. I'd watch celebrity chefs on TV and feel like I couldn't do that. Finding my own kitchen cure made me feel capable. I learned to cook food with purpose. If your kids are sick, you can go to the kitchen and make a soup for your babies to give them something healing beyond Motrin. Food goes to the root—your digestive system.
>
> My kids watched me get well. My own mother was helpless to her disease, unfortunately. I didn't realize what it meant to be the child of an ill parent, and I realized that I was living that legacy and passing it on to my own children. Now I've shifted their emotional inheritance.
>
> The kitchen is a great place to find yourself. But these days, we're not in our homes much. We believe in convenience and are just coming out of a phase where cooking was often regarded as a waste of time. We were busy consuming and buying things outside, so we lost our relationship with our home. When you lose your relationship with your home, you lose the relationship with your life.
>
> Getting into the kitchen is a great way to root and ground yourself. When I'm spread out energetically, I say

to myself, *I'll go to the kitchen today. Chopping is my meditation.* Everyone in the family feeds off the mother, and she needs a place to ground herself and become balanced. Sitting down at your own table to eat is so important.

Mee's healing foods are very specific to her own autoimmune disease, which gives her quick feedback. She told me that she turned a corner when she started to eat mineral-rich sea vegetables. Collard greens, kale, leafy greens, bok choy, cabbage, and brussels sprouts are also healing for her. But she made a very important discovery: She has to rotate the foods that she eats.

Mee's husband, Lee McCormick, owns a grass-fed cattle ranch. "Just like the cows have to rotate through different pastures because they need a variety of grasses, we also need variety," Mee told me.

"Most people eat the same things all the time and may develop low-grade food allergies to them," she added. So Mee rotates her burdock and carrots, sweet potatoes, squashes, and winter veggies—all packed with fiber. She drinks aloe-vera juice to heal ulcerations and drinks cabbage juice to feed her probiotic bacteria. Mee also eats beans and grains, always carefully soaked to remove the antinutrients. Millet, quinoa, amaranth, and brown rice are healing foods for her; and lentils are the best of all legumes. They move well through her digestive tract.

While dairy isn't right for Mee, pasture-raised eggs are. You can read more about her healing journey and sample some wonderful recipes in her book, *My Kitchen Cure.* Fortunately for us all, Mee allowed me to include several of her recipes in Chapter 27.

Josh and Keith

I've mentioned my friends Josh and Keith. Josh is a handsome guy, a holistic health coach who works in a traditional Chinese and integrative-medicine practice. A big guy at 6'3", he weighed 295 pounds before switching to the PlantPlus way. In seven months, he dropped to 240 pounds, and now he's a slim and vibrant 220.

Here's his account of how he did it, along with his partner Keith's story. An acupuncturist, Keith lost 25 pounds in the same time frame. When two people in the same family go PlantPlus together, they get the benefit of inspiring each other, of course. How did Josh and Keith do it? Josh explained:

> I had resigned myself to being a big guy, gaining weight and being fat forever. But the first thing that Keith and I did was cut out grains and beans. That was much easier than I expected. I didn't eat a lot of bread to begin with, but I did eat a lot of pasta whenever we ate out.
>
> Then I became the omelet master. They're so easy to make, and they fill you up. After two weeks, I noticed that my inflammation was gone—the daily joint achiness and muscle soreness disappeared. And I had far less gas. When the constant bloat in my gut went away, that felt great. No more baby bump. I didn't work out for the first ten weeks because I was so heavy that it was just too hard. And I had no motivation.
>
> But the weight just fell off. It happened in stages. For a week or two or three, nothing would happen, and then I'd lose five pounds. I also try not to get on the scale too much. Inches lost and how I feel are more important to me.
>
> Losing the weight has been pretty effortless. I haven't missed anything or felt deprived. Keith and I give ourselves one cheat day a week, but usually, it's just one meal. We don't use the cheat day much because eating food that makes you feel bad isn't worth it. Even popcorn at a movie makes me feel bloated.
>
> Keith makes a lot of smoothies with kale or arugula, cilantro, parsley—any kind of greens. He adds a little fruit and a handful of nuts, and maybe some avocado and coconut oil.
>
> For lunch at work, we have salads from a local deli. I might even eat two of them. I eat at least three servings of greens for lunch every day. Even some fast-food places have great salads when we're in a hurry. I actually *crave*

vegetables. I never thought that would happen! Sautéed kale sounds very good these days.

Keith's grandmother makes great collards, and she inspired us. Now we sauté kale or chard a lot. We use a little water with vinegar or lemon juice in the bottom of the pan, and sauté the greens until half of them change color—about ten minutes. Then we let them sit, or we eat them right away. We have a Misto to spray our own olive oil. Using that means that you can coat the greens and not use a ton of oil. We like to add some Bragg Liquid Aminos and throw in shredded carrots to cut the bitterness. A little raw apple-cider vinegar is great, too. It gives the greens a slighty spicy kick. Sometimes we add flavor with garlic and onion or radishes (regular or daikon) that we shred with a hand grater.

Cauliflower is a staple in our house—it's heaven sent. You can do so much with it. It's the perfect filler. Some nights we spray cauliflower, broccoli, or brussels sprouts with olive oil; add a bit of salt and pepper; and then roast them at 400 degrees until they're slightly charred. We love crunchiness, and it's so easy. Then we might make a bed of fresh arugula on our plates, and top that with some meat and the roasted veggies. It's great to put extra raw greens on your plate.

I also make a lot of slaws. My favorite starts with a package of broccoli slaw (cauliflower and broccoli stems—about an inch long and thin—that have been shredded). To that I add some cabbage, cilantro, green onion, cucumber, and shredded carrot. I mix it with about half a cup of apple-cider vinegar, some Bragg's, a little salt-free seasoning mix, and maybe a touch of cayenne. I mix that up good and let it sit in the fridge for a day. To serve, I top it with a bit of olive oil. It's my late snack now, instead of ice cream. The sour flavor helped me beat my sweet cravings.

Most of the time, we prepare meats simply, using a frying pan or grill pan. We always use some kind of marinade—olive oil; lemon or lime; or vinegar with different spices, herbs, garlic, or onion. Or sometimes herbes de Provence. The marinade starts to break the meat down. We haven't breaded anything at home and haven't missed it. We save that for cheat days. We wanted to avoid the feeling of replacing anything and focus on doing new things.

We snack on slaws and lots of raw nuts. Target carries raw mixed nuts—you can get a giant container for about 12 bucks. But I don't always have to snack if I get a decent amount of protein at meals. My blood sugar doesn't go crazy.

The PlantPlus Diet is very mood stabilizing. My friends used to joke, "Josh is getting hungry—we better feed him before he eats one of us!" I was known for going a little crazy if I got too hungry.

The biggest change for Keith and me is that we cook way more. We've saved a lot of money and finally put some away in an IRA. The diet has even been good for our dogs. Sassy, our English bulldog, was really overweight. Last year she had an allergic reaction to something and spent three nights at the emergency vet. Now, our dogs eat grain-free food. Sassy went from 55 to 40 pounds. Her alopecia (hair loss) has almost cleared up, and she acts like a puppy at eight years old. She'd never eat a carrot before. Now she'll eat carrots and broccoli stems as treats.

Personalization: Your Own Evolving PlantPlus Story

I hope that the journeys of my colleagues and co-conspirators have inspired you. Sharing your own story with a buddy who's also on the path to better health can definitely inspire you both. It's fascinating how interesting food can be when you're engaged in a conscious relationship with it. Observing how your body

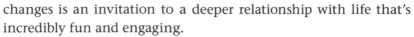

changes is an invitation to a deeper relationship with life that's incredibly fun and engaging.

Congratulations are in order when you've completed your four-week Reboot. Then it's time to take stock of the results and decide whether you want to reintroduce some of the foods you eliminated. Here's what to do:

1. **Revisit your test scores:** If you asked your doc for the tests that we discussed in Chapter 18, or if you're being treated for health problems, you already have a baseline for comparison. You'll want to know if the Reboot made a positive difference or not. So see your doc, and have the tests done again.

2. **Do a self-assessment:** Review your diary, get on the scale, and retake the Medical Symptom Checklist that you filled out before the Reboot. Compare the new one to the old one. How are you doing?

3. **Try a food challenge:** After the Reboot, my husband, Gordon—who adores New Mexican cuisine—was missing beans and looking forward to making some chili. We decided to try a food challenge. That means eating a normal-size portion of the food in question, along with your usual foods. *Important: Reintroduce only one food at a time, and wait at least three days before you try it again or before you initiate a challenge with a different food.*

Pinto beans were the first food we attempted to add back to our diet. The result was immediate in terms of the fabled flatulence that makes beans such a hit with kids. But in addition to the gas, I felt "off" for the rest of the day. By "off," I mean continuously bloated, achy, and lethargic. The result of reintroducing the pinto beans was *malaise*—a term generally used by doctors to describe the feeling tone of illness. Gordon, on the other hand, felt just fine, thank you.

We did another bean challenge a few weeks later with kidney beans. Gordon once again felt fine. But me? Not so much. In retrospect, I might have done better if I soaked the beans in water for several hours and then cooked them, which removes some of the lectins and antinutrients. But hey. We live at almost 9,000 feet, and up here, canned beans are what you get. I tried to make pea soup once. It simmered for nearly two days, and the peas never got soft. They resembled BBs. Red lentils, on the other hand, cook very quickly. I can eat small quantities of those (maybe a quarter cup in a bowl of soup) and do just fine.

I tried one more legume experiment with garbanzo beans, also known as chickpeas. We bought a tub of locally produced, whole-food, organic hummus, which is abundantly available here in Boulder, Colorado. I can eat a small amount of that without any noticeable problems either.

Emboldened by that discovery, I bought a bag of chickpea flour, long used by Europeans to make pizza crusts. But a single piece of chickpea pizza did me in: malaise, fatigue, bloating, and cramps. But chickpea flour also makes great tortillas. Since the tortillas are paper thin, I can get away with eating a small one, but I generally don't since the thought of exceeding my limit makes the idea less than appealing. I've included a recipe for these tasty chickpea tortillas, though, in case they agree with you.

What about grains? We've continued to eliminate grains from our diet (for the most part) because I can't think of any good reason to include them except for the rare slice of pizza (once in a blue moon) on a night out. In spite of all the press about healthy whole grains, they're not as nutrient dense as most of the vegetables and fruits that we eat. So why add the carbs, the calories, the lectins, and the endless temptation of flour-based foods?

Mindful Eating

Because keeping a food diary for a few months trains you to pay attention to the nuances of bodily sensation, you start to tune in more reliably to what your body needs and what upsets it.

Mindfulness is about paying attention—just noticing—without interpreting, judging, rationalizing, or getting emotionally entangled in whatever you're observing. So instead of noticing that you're bloated and calling yourself stupid for eating something that made you feel bad, you just notice, *Oh, those beans didn't agree with me. That's interesting.*

Mindfulness, as you already know, is also the secret of pleasure. Wolfing down a square or two of dark chocolate mindlessly, for example, isn't much fun. But when you let it melt in your mouth slowly, savoring the way that it coats your tongue, how the saliva rises to greet it, the way it slides down your throat, and how the aftertaste lingers, the pleasure is practically orgasmic. While less romantic, mindfully eating onions or berries, greens or nuts, chicken or fish, tofu or tempeh, can give you a lot of pleasure, too.

Increasing mindfulness of how different foods affect your metabolism is an ongoing process for life. Your body, and the foods it requires, may change with aging, pregnancy, stress, illness, antibiotic use, or in response to moving to—or even visiting—a different climate. Staying tuned in to your inner-information channel will help you adjust to new circumstances without gaining weight or compromising your health.

Live and Let Live

Back in the 1970s, when I was an assistant professor of anatomy and cell biology at Tufts Medical School, a young man in his 20s named Aaron slouched listlessly into my laboratory one day. How he got there is still a mystery. Aaron was wan and thin. His hair was falling out and so were his teeth. He had come looking for answers as to why that was so, especially since he took great pains with his diet.

"What do you eat?" I asked. He replied that he ate only fruits, sprouts, tree nuts, and leafy vegetables. In the spring and summer, he ate his vegetables raw, but in the winter, he cooked them in a little olive oil.

"Do you eat tofu or tempeh?" I asked. "Grains or beans? Tubers?"

He shook his head to the negative. "No, I eat only the most evolved foods—vegetables and fruits that grow above ground or hang from trees. I'm on a spiritual journey and want to eat foods that support my expanding consciousness."

Spirituality, I explained, is all about mindfulness and compassion. Starving himself and destroying his health was neither mindful nor compassionate. Aaron obviously needed protein, fat, and some starchy carbs as well. He was a sweet guy and took the feedback he'd asked for with grace, but decided to stick to his diet anyway since he was convinced that it was the fast track to enlightenment.

If you believe in reincarnation, perhaps that's true. But in his current body, Aaron wasn't going to get too far.

Since he wasn't intent on converting other people to his largely fruitarian ways, Aaron was harmless to them even though he was clearly a menace to himself. But that's not the case with some diet fundamentalists, whose opinions trump both mindfulness and kindness.

I was cruising the Huffington Post Healthy Living Section one day and came across an interesting video with this header: "Alexandra Jamieson, co-creator of *Super Size Me,* joins HuffPost Live to discuss why she quit being a vegan" (http://live.huffingtonpost .com/r/archive/segment/former-vegan-i-am-never-defining-how-i -eat-ever-again/529e3ac378c90a10e900014a). She spoke about why "I am never defining how I eat ever again."

After ten years as a vegan, with a couple of books about the vegan lifestyle under her belt and an active lecturing and coaching schedule, Alex spoke very humbly about feeling sick, craving meat, and then feeling deeply ashamed.

For a while she lived two lives—sneaking out to eat animal foods while pretending to be a vegan. What a painful, but ultimately freeing experience both for herself and her followers. By paying attention to her body and its needs, she added eggs, fish, and meat to her plant-based diet. In being true to herself and to her own metabolism, her health improved.

I went to her website and found an open letter she had written about her shift in diet (http://alexandrajamieson.com/im -not-vegan-anymore). It was heartening to read the comments of people who applauded her honesty and decision to honor what her body needed. It was shocking, though, to see the number of hostile comments that were discounting, hateful, and thoroughly lacking in compassion. In the HuffPo interview, Alex revealed that she had even received death threats. How ironic. In the name of compassion for animals, there are folks out there who would contemplate killing a human being.

When the Dalai Lama was asked why he still eats meat when he believes in *ahimsa,* or "no harm," his reply was that his body needs it. And so it is for some of us.

There's a new word called *orthorexia*—an eating disorder that centers on thinking that we have to eat just right. For that reason alone, I think that having a "cheat" meal once a week or so after the Reboot is over (*always out of your home*) is a good idea. It helps prevent hardening of the attitude and hopefully discourages judgment of yourself and others.

One year when I was a speaker at a major health expo, I watched a famous alkaline-diet guru polish off a huge plate of french fries with obvious relish. *Good on him,* I thought. He eats well, but he's not a fundamentalist. So if you see me walking down the street licking an ice-cream cone on a hot summer's day, please celebrate my flexibility rather than punish my lack of rigidity. And do the same for yourself.

∅ ∅ ∅

This concludes your tour of the Reboot and Personalization stages of the PlantPlus Diet. I've kept things simple, which will hopefully make it easier for you to get on board with your new lifestyle.

In the next and final section of the book, I'll provide a list of Superfoods for you to incorporate into your PlantPlus Diet plan, suitable both for the Reboot and for later Personalization. When you eat delicious food that's in balance with your own personal metabolic fingerprint, you'll be amazed by how easily you can lose weight and regain health and vitality. Then we'll get to the recipes that I hope you've been waiting for.

PART IV

LET'S EAT!

We'll begin this section with a tour of my favorite Superfoods so that you can understand why so many of them appear in the recipes. Then we'll discuss how to eat well for less. That chapter will explain why I've included recipes that will feed you for several meals at lower cost.

Finally . . . the recipes. One of my students e-mailed me a year ago, excited that I was writing a cookbook. Well, *not exactly,* I wrote back. There's a lot of other stuff in the book, too.

I thank you for your willingness to absorb all this information before you've even tasted my cooking! I've included some practical weights and measures in the recipe section for those of you who haven't been in the kitchen lately. I hope it's fun for you to get back in there if you've gone missing for a while.

We'll conclude with one final chapter, "PlantPlus Lite"—a simple way to start your journey if you're not yet ready for the whole enchilada of Reboot and Personalization.

CHAPTER 25

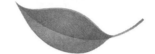

Dr. Joan's 20 Superfoods

*"Eat an apple on going to bed, and you'll
keep the doctor from earning his bread."*

— FEBRUARY 1866 EDITION OF *NOTES AND QUERIES* MAGAZINE

Are there really foods with proven healing properties? I think we all know a few of these—from apples to chicken soup. My mother always made chicken soup when someone in the family was ill, and recent research has indeed shown that bone broth has antiviral properties. Herbs and spices used for millennia to improve health and mood, once dismissed as old wives' tales, are now the subject of modern research.

For example, my favorite medicinal food for colds, flus, and stomach viruses is ginger, which we now know is a powerful anti-inflammatory and antioxidant. A related subterranean rhizome called turmeric contains *curcumin* that increases brain-derived neurotrophic factor (BDNF), which stimulates the growth of new neurons and helps prevent Alzheimer's disease.

In this chapter, I'll introduce you to some common Super-foods that are useful for a variety of reasons—both medicinal and nutritional. Some, like nuts, are portable and supersatiating—they stop hunger and give you needed protein, fat, and micronutrients. Others have specific qualities that counteract the Five Pillars of Dietary Doom you read about in Chapter 2. They reduce oxidative stress, inflammation, and glycation, as well as provide micronutrients and fiber to keep the gut flora healthy and diverse. When we get to my PlantPlus recipes in the next chapter, you'll know *why* I've featured all these delicious Superfoods in them. And when you create your own meals, you'll have these fantastic ingredients in mind.

Dr. Joan's Favorite Superfoods

Please note: These Superfoods are in no particular order.

1. Nuts and Seeds

During the Reboot and early months of PlantPlus when you're losing weight and adjusting your metabolism, nuts are very important foods. A handful (a quarter cup) is very satiating, and many diet docs recommend eating a quarter cup twice a day—as a morning and an afternoon snack if you feel the need. But as fine a food as nuts are, they still have a lot of calories, so more than two quarter-cup portions a day can stall weight loss.

Almonds, cashews, walnuts, pecans, pistachios, hazelnuts, macadamias, and sunflower seeds can be eaten daily. But watch out for peanuts (actually legumes), which are often contaminated with a fungus that can cause liver cancer. Brazil nuts also deserve special mention. They're the most concentrated dietary source of the trace element selenium, a critical cofactor for the all-important antioxidant enzymes *glutathione peroxidase* and *thioredoxin reductase*. One nut gives you all the selenium you need for the day. But more may push the limits of selenium toxicity, especially if you habitually overindulge. One ounce (six to eight nuts) gives you 544 micrograms (mcg) of selenium, ten times more than the recommended daily allowance of 55 mcg per day.

A few health benefits: Nuts are rich in fiber to help keep you feeling full and to feed your probiotic gut bacteria. They're also rich in L-arginine, which makes artery walls more flexible and less prone to blood clots. A good source of vitamin E, they are also rich in antioxidants. Both Gordon and I have cardiologists who wax poetic over the cardiovascular benefit of nuts.

A note on soaking nuts and seeds: While soaking raw nuts helps remove bitter tannins, enzyme inhibitors, and antinutrient phytates that interfere with the absorption of vitamins and minerals, use your own judgment about soaking. You can buy presoaked nuts and seeds at many health-food stores; soak, dry, and roast them yourself; or get them on the Internet at sources like natesrawharvest.com. Blue Mountain Organics (www .bluemountainorganics.com/betterthanroasted) also has a high-quality line of presoaked roasted nuts and nut butters.

We like MaraNatha brand organic roasted or raw nut butters. They're not presoaked as far as I know, but they're delicious and they sit just fine with Gordon and me. The problem with commercial nuts is more than the antinutrients, however. I was starved one day while out doing errands—the very reason why it's good to carry snacks with you—and bought a package of mixed nuts at the gas station. Sure enough, they were cooked in cottonseed oil. Ugh! Cotton, which isn't a food, is the most pesticide-laden crop in the world. The moral of the story is to read the label before you buy the nuts.

2. Nut Flour

One of the great delights of a PlantPlus Diet are the nut-based baked goods. Even on your Reboot, you can enjoy my about-to-be-famous chocolate-chip cookies, coconut-bliss cookies, or thumbprint cookies—substituting two or three cookies for a quarter-cup serving of nuts. You can also enjoy my delectable almond-and-flaxseed-meal breads (one slice substitutes for a quarter cup of whole nuts), and roasted sesame crackers or seed crackers.

Most health-food stores carry Bob's Red Mill organic nut flours (I generally use almond flour, but occasionally add in some hazelnut for extra punch). Bob's Red Mill works well enough for most cookies and has the advantage of being available in bulk at our local Costco, which saves a few bucks.

My preferred almond flour, however, comes from Honeyville Farms. I purchase it online at http://shop.honeyville.com /blanched-almond-flour.html. The blanched-almond flour is lower in phytates and ground very fine, which gives bread a superior texture. Since you won't be eating carloads of baked goods, the flour—though costly—goes a long way. It will keep in your refrigerator for about six months.

3. Yogurt and Fermented Foods

Aim for eating two servings of fermented foods daily, as microbiologists exploring the world of a healthy microbiome suggest. We almost always start the day with a yogurt-berry shake or Greek yogurt mixed with thawed frozen berries or sliced and crushed fresh berries that create a nice juicy mix. Sauerkraut is also a favorite in our home. Just a few tablespoons as a relish does the trick. We learned to ferment our own sauerkraut—very simple and supercheap. If you buy sauerkraut, kimchi, or other fermented foods, look in the refrigerated section of the store since pasteurization or canning kills the probiotics.

4. Apples

In 2004, the USDA checked the antioxidant levels in over 100 antioxidant-rich foods. Granny Smith apples ranked 13th. Eating an apple a day may also slow weight gain, since apples contain a type of fiber that encourages the growth of Bacteroidetes bacteria (the thin makers) over Firmicutes (the thrifty fat makers).

The peels contain a disease-fighting class of phytochemicals known as *triterpenoids*, which are being evaluated for use in treating breast cancer and preventing its recurrence.[1] Triterpenoids occur naturally in various plants—seaweeds, apples, cranberries, figs, olives, lavender, oregano, rosemary, and thyme. These phytochemicals retard growth of cancer cells in the liver, colon, and other sites as well as the breast.[2]

Triterpenoids are also anti-inflammatory agents. Among other benefits, they reduce oxidative stress, regulate the cell cycle, inhibit cell proliferation, and help repair mutations in the genetic code.

Apples help in the blood-sugar department as well. As you know, they're rich in fiber, which curbs blood-sugar swings. They also contain a phytochemical called *quercetin* that inhibits the enzymes that break complex carbs down into simple sugars. An apple can level out your blood sugar and prevent spikes, keeping you feeling full for longer. In addition, apples stimulate the beta cells of the pancreas to secrete insulin, and they also stimulate insulin receptors so that more glucose is taken up into the cells and there's less glucose on the loose to create AGEs.

A recent study out of the Department of Nutrition at the Harvard School for Public Health looked at data from three cohorts of health professionals. Although this was an observational study, it showed that eating different types of fruit correlated with reduction in the risk of developing type 2 diabetes. Eating three servings weekly of apples, blueberries, pears, grapes, or raisins all reduced the apparent incidence of diabetes by 7 percent. Drinking the juice of these fruits, however, correlated with an increased risk of diabetes.[3]

5. Chocolate

Cacao, the ancient Aztec food of the gods, is nutrient dense and packed with antioxidants that sop up the tissue-damaging free radicals that cause aging. The phytonutrients in cacao can also help lower blood pressure, fight atherosclerosis, and reduce the risk of stroke. And as many women agree, chocolate has a romantic feel to it. Perhaps that's because it contains PEA (*phenethylamine*), a neurohormone released when you're in love—or at least infatuated. PEA, in turn, releases happy-making endorphins. The flavonoids in chocolate even reduce insulin resistance, and since dark chocolate has a low-glycemic index, a tablespoon or two of organic, low-sugar hot fudge, or a few squares of an eco-friendly dark-chocolate bar, won't cause spikes in your blood sugar.

Dark chocolate (55 percent or more cacao) is relatively bitter, so it's less tempting to overeat than sweet milk chocolate. I love the story behind Alter Eco dark organic almond bars, and eat them frequently. They're 60 percent cacao, harvested from the Acopagro Co-op in Ecuador on the edge of the Peruvian Amazon. In 1994 a United Nations program helped the farmers there make the switch from growing coca for the dangerous drug trade to growing cacao trees that are now part of a large project to restore the rain forest canopy.

Just for fun, let's take a look at an Alter Eco chocolate bar and see what else—other than being dark and fair trade—makes it a good fit for PlantPlus. Whenever you buy chocolate, you can do this same kind of analysis: Is it good for you, and is it good for the environment?

One Alter Eco chocolate almond bar weighs 2.82 ounces and consists of 10 large, flat sections. One serving (listed on the label as 5 sections) contains 220 calories, 19 grams of carbs (14 of them sugar), and 4 grams of fiber, for a net carb count of 15—about the same as a medium apple. I've never actually eaten 5 whole squares at a sitting. One or two pieces, eaten slowly (for maximum enjoyment, eat chocolate mindfully—snapping off tiny bits and letting them melt in your mouth), are a very healthful and satisfying treat with very little sugar and few carbs.

6. Avocados

These creamy green fruits are rich in fiber (10 grams per fruit). Since feeding our gut microbes is always on my mind (well, not exactly *always*), avocados are frequently on the menu.

Our resident microbes need a wide variety of fiber, and avocados contain both soluble and insoluble types. The insoluble fiber not only feeds your microbes but also moves food residue through the gut (think regularity). The soluble fiber keeps you feeling full for a long time since it forms a gel, combining with water in the tummy. Avocados are also a source of good fat, predominantly monounsaturated fat similar to what's found in olive oil. As a bonus, avocado oil has an unusually high smoke point and is a great choice when you want a neutral-flavored oil for cooking or baking.

7. Berries

Berries—from blueberries to boysenberries, strawberries to blackberries, cranberries to raspberries—are Superfoods. Fresh or frozen, their health powers remain intact. While berries can be expensive, our local Costco sells large bags of premium organic frozen berries at a very reasonable price. Frozen berries are convenient and available year-round. That's what we use in our morning yogurt-berry smoothies, berry sauces, and baked goods. We also enjoy berries fresh, of course.

Berries are low in calories and high in fiber, and they won't make your blood sugar soar. They're also rich in antioxidant flavonoids. An article in *Scientific American* titled "Your Brain on Blueberries: Enhance Memory with the Right Foods" reviewed some of the research concerning berries and cognitive function:

Emerging research suggests that compounds in blueberries known as flavonoids may improve memory, learning and general cognitive function, including reasoning skills, decision making, verbal comprehension and numerical ability. In addition, studies comparing dietary habits with cognitive function in adults hint that consuming flavonoids may help slow the decline in mental facility that is often seen with aging and might even provide protection against disorders such as Alzheimer's and Parkinson's.[4]

Personally I'd eat berries just for the flavor, even if they weren't such a great source of flavonoids. Cranberries, among other health benefits, can stop bacteria from attaching to the lining of the urinary tract and causing UTIs (urinary tract infections)—a chronic health problem for many women. This tart red berry can also prevent the *H. pylori* bacteria from attaching to the wall of the stomach and causing ulcers. And as an added benefit, a compound isolated from cranberries helps prevent plaque formation on the teeth.

8. Coffee, Black Tea, White Tea, and Green Tea

Here's reason to rejoice (at least if you love coffee or tea). Coffee and tea are health foods—a verdict that has emerged from years of controversial research. Coffee is the single most important source of antioxidants for Americans. And tea, while less popular than coffee in America, is the most frequently consumed beverage in the world, after water.

While different herbal teas have their own healing properties (a book in itself), and many of them are caffeine-free, they're made from roots, flowers, spices, and herbs that don't contain the flavonoids that come from the leaves of the plant *Camellia sinensis*, which are harvested and processed to become either black, green, or white tea.

> Coffee may lower the risk of type 2 diabetes, colon cancer, Parkinson's disease, and gout. But if you have high blood pressure, anxiety, a sleep disturbance, or a mood disorder, choose water-processed (not chemically processed) decaf.

A word of caution. While tea and coffee are noncaloric, adding a lot of cream, sweetened soymilk, sugar, artificial flavoring, and syrups can turn these drinks into chemical concoctions and caloric disasters. For example, a Starbucks pumpkin-spice latte (12 ounces) has 240 calories, roughly the same as a candy bar. A 16-ounce grande will put you back 310 calories. And don't forget that all that sugar will AGE you.

9. Eggs from Free-Range Chickens

After years of us being told not to eat eggs because of their high cholesterol content, the tide has finally turned. Even the most conservative guidelines from the American Heart Association give the green light to an egg a day. And a lot of experts think that even an egg a day is a very conservative number.

David Katz, M.D., director of the Yale Prevention Research Center, "eggsonerated" eggs in a delightful HuffPo article entitled "Unscrambling Egg Science." He performed some much-needed surgery on a piece of observational research (conducted by a vegan, by the way) that compared eating eggs to smoking cigarettes, a study that unfortunately left egg on an otherwise fine researcher's face.

> Katz gave eggs a resounding not-guilty verdict, citing evidence from his own lab and others' that dietary cholesterol is "mostly, if not entirely, innocuous, when isolated from the company it often keeps in the diet."

Katz went on to put eggs into a highly sensible evolutionary context:

> . . . while saturated fat intake in the Stone Age was next to nil, cholesterol intake from both eggs and organ meats of hunted animals was substantial. It is, in a word, illogical that the human body would be harmed by something to which it is long adapted. It would be a bit like concluding that wildebeest is harmful for lions; bamboo is bad for pandas. Eggs have been part of the "native" human diet since long before the advent of the first domesticated chicken. Science is generally at its best when bounded by sense.[5]

I was deeply touched when Katz talked about the fact that he'd given up eggs for 20 years because he didn't like how hens were treated on factory farms. Now, however, he's added humanely produced organic, free-range, local eggs back into his diet. If you're going to eat eggs, please buy the latter. Yes, they're more expensive than the factory-farmed kind, but overall they're still a very economical source of protein and micronutrients.

10. Ginger Root

Ginger is a rhizome or subterranean stem that comes from a plant belonging to the family *Zingiberaceae* (yes, it sure is zingy). We always have a bag of these knobby rhizomes in our refrigerator, since eating ginger is a big part of our daily anti-inflammatory regime. It's delicious in sauces, marinades, teas, and smoothies.

> Ginger has broad anti-inflammatory effects mediated by well-researched pathways that spare the body the side effects of commercial nonsteroidal anti-inflammatory drugs (NSAIDs). Ginger actually inhibits the induction of several genes involved in the inflammatory response.[6]

This magnificent root has been used medicinally for thousands of years to curb nausea and vomiting, and for a diversity of other gastrointestinal symptoms ranging from flatulence to colic. These days it's often recommended to alleviate nausea in patients receiving chemo, for inflammatory conditions like arthritis pain, and for colds and cough. One teaspoon of grated ginger simmered with eight ounces of water—with a little bit of honey and lemon—is very soothing for colds and sore throats. We use ginger root—along with its relative, turmeric root—in our delicious smoothies.

11. Bhakti Chai

This off-the-charts beverage combines the health benefits of black tea, fresh-pressed ginger, and other fresh spices—all organically sourced and nonGMO—with superior taste and laudable social responsibility. Although I have no vested interest in any of the other products I recommend in this book, I do have an interest in Bhakti Chai. I'm a friend of Brook Eddy, the young entrepreneur (a single mom of twins, no less), who founded and oversees the company. She lived in my home for a while in the pre–Bhakti Chai days when we were both single. I'm proud to be an investor in her dream.

Brook founded Bhakti Chai in 2006, inspired by the chai she tasted in India a few years before. Her chai is amazingly rich and spicy—a taste that most people find addictive in the best sense of the word. *Bhakti,* Brook explains, means "devotion through social action" in Sanskrit. A portion of her profits go to improve the lives of women worldwide, including grants to social-activist entrepreneurs. And the chai is too good for words. It has won numerous awards ranging from Best Chai in Best of Boulder, to Best Chai Tea in the Taster's Choice Awards reviewed in the *San Francisco Chronicle,* to the coveted SOFI Gold award in New York City for Outstanding Hot Beverage, and more.

Here's the welcome message at www.bhaktichai.com:

> Bhakti Chai infuses fresh-pressed organic ginger and fiery spices into Fair Trade Certified black tea for a chai that energizes the spirit. Bhakti Chai comes in both a concentrate that can be blended with any variety of milk or non-dairy beverage at a 1:1 ratio, and as Iced Bhakti Chai, available pre-mixed with organic, nonGMO soy in 16-ounce, ready-to-drink glass bottles. Both can be found in the dairy case or the refrigerated beverage aisle at grocery stores nationwide.

We buy unsweetened Bhakti Chai. That way we can use a little stevia for sweetening and mix the chai with almond- or soymilk. For me, a cup of Bhakti Chai is like dessert.

12. Turmeric

This Superfood (*Curcuma longa*) is a root that, like ginger, is a powerful antioxidant and anti-inflammatory used medicinally for thousands of years. Turmeric is rich in *curcumin* (5 to 10 percent of the root), a yellow plant pigment or phytonutrient that's been shown to increase brain levels of a hormone that stimulates the growth of neurons—brain-derived neurotrophic factor (BDNF).

Since elderly villagers in India have practically no Alzheimer's disease, epidemiologists took note. What's the reason? Genes, diet, or both? Traditionally, Indian villagers eat curries rich in turmeric at most meals. The curcumin dissolves in the cooking fat, which increases its bioavailability. That's important, since if you can't absorb or make use of a nutrient, it doesn't matter how much you ingest. That's the problem with many supplements.

For a comprehensive article on curcumin, whether or not it's bioavailable as a supplement, and the current state of research, go to http://alzheimer.neurology.ucla.edu/Curcumin.html.

I use the raw root along with ginger in yogurt smoothies and add powdered turmeric to almond bread, mixing it into the butter or coconut oil that's part of the recipe. You can't taste the turmeric, but it gives the bread a wonderful, earthy, warm-yellow color. We add powdered turmeric to stir-fries, soups, marinades, and stews as well.

13. Cardamom

Another plant in the ginger family, cardamom produces small pods containing seeds. Either whole or ground into powder, the seeds give Indian food an aromatic, enchanting, exotic flavor. Like ginger, cardamom has a long history of medicinal use for gastrointestinal problems, arthritis, and respiratory problems. It also has powerful anti-inflammatory and antioxidant properties.

Cardamom is my favorite of all spices. I use it in cappuccino, spike stewed fruits with it, put it in gelatin desserts, and generally turn into putty in its presence. It's a strong taste, and while some people love it, others—like Gordon—care for it only when used in moderation.

14. Cinnamon

There are several varieties of cinnamon, which is the inner bark of a tree. Another medicinal herb that's been used for thousands of years, it's also one of the world's most popular spices. One of the benefits of cinnamon is that it mimics the effects of insulin and may improve blood-glucose control. The abstract from a 2010 review article summarizes some of the research:

> The available . . . evidence suggests that cinnamon has anti-inflammatory, antimicrobial, antioxidant, antitumor, cardiovascular, cholesterol-lowering, and immunomodulatory effects. In

vitro studies have demonstrated that cinnamon may act as an insulin mimetic, to potentiate insulin activity or to stimulate cellular glucose metabolism. . . . The use of cinnamon as an adjunct to the treatment of type 2 diabetes mellitus is the most promising area, but further research is needed before definitive recommendations can be made.[7]

My recommendation is to use cinnamon liberally, because it makes food so delicious and the house so fragrant. I add it to smoothies, baked apples, cookies, coffee, stewed fruits, and, sometimes, almond bread if I'm making a sweet, rather than a savory, loaf.

15. Chili Peppers

Yes, indeed, some like it hot. The phytochemical *capsaicin* is what gives jalapeños, habaneros, chipotles, cayenne, and other chili peppers their heat. Capsaicin is useful in relieving pain—you can even get it in topical cream formulations—because it releases endorphins. It also lowers blood pressure and gives metabolism a mild boost, which helps with weight maintenance. Recent research confirms that capsaicin lowers LDL cholesterol by increasing its excretion. It also blocks the action of a gene that causes arteries to contract, raising blood pressure and reducing blood flow to tissues. By lowering blood pressure and relaxing arteries, capsaicin is helpful to heart health.[8]

Hot Indian curries make ample use of chili powder. Fortunately, they're traditionally served with yogurt sauce or *raita*. The milk protein neutralizes capsaicin and cuts the heat—just in case you need to know. If you're processing hot peppers at home (even relatively mild jalapeños), be sure to wear rubber gloves. The capsaicin from the membranes and seeds lingers on the skin, and if you rub your eyes, even hours later, you'll feel the burn.

Gordon loves hot curries, hot peppers, and hot sauce. We have a wide variety ranging from Tabasco to imported Thai and Mexican specialty sauces. If you love hot sauce, be sure to read the label since some of them contain quite a bit of sugar.

16. Sardines

Look for either fresh or canned sardines. These little fish are low on the food chain and therefore low in pollutants like mercury that accumulate in larger fish that eat smaller ones, thus concentrating the toxins in their own fat. Sardines are wild caught rather than farmed and are rich in vital omega-3 fatty acids. Gordon loves canned sardines (and the dogs love the juice). Because they are so convenient, he can put them on a salad and have a tasty meal in a jiffy. Alas, I never learned to like sardines. My loss.

But perhaps, as with Gordon, they're a Superfood for you.

17. Chicken Soup

When you make a chicken or turkey soup and boil the bones, the resulting broth contains gelatin and thickens when it's refrigerated. Gelatin is actually the *collagen* that comes from the bones and connective tissue of the bird. Bone broth has been used as a folk medicine for thousands of years and is an important component of traditional diets, including Paleo diets and ethnic diets. Recent research shows that chicken soup really does reduce cold symptoms.[9]

18. Extra-Virgin Olive Oil (EVOO)

Olive oil, as I mentioned in Chapter 6, "Cherish Good Fats," is a Superfood. Let me reiterate a few highlights from that discussion: EVOO is a monounsaturated fatty acid (MUFA), so it's more stable and less prone to oxidation than the PUFAs. A Mediterranean diet, arguably one of the healthiest diets overall, is rich both in olive oil and in omega-3s from seafood. In addition to being healthful, fine olive oil is intoxicatingly fragrant and delicious. It adds a subtle, sweet-earthy flavor to whatever foods you add it to.

People who consume olive oil as a regular part of their diet are less likely to develop cardiovascular disease, including stroke, high blood pressure, high cholesterol levels, and high triglycerides.

Olive oil also helps preserve the endothelial layer (the inside lining) of blood vessels and reduce inflammation, which may be part of the way it prevents the buildup of plaque and fights hardening of the arteries.

Olive oil is also high in a substance called hydroxytyrosol, which is being explored at Houston Methodist Cancer Center as a preventative for breast cancer in a high-risk group of women. The MUFAs in EVOO also help regularize carbohydrate metabolism and dampen down spikes in blood sugar.

19. Kale

This nutrient-dense, dark, leafy green is often referred to as the "queen of greens." It's a member of the Brassica family of cruciferous vegetables, which includes cabbage, cauliflower, collards, brussels sprouts, and broccoli. All cruciferous vegetables have anticancer properties. In addition, kale is especially rich in vitamins A, C, and K (all antioxidants); fiber; and a range of micronutrients, including copper, manganese, and phosphorus. It can help lower blood pressure and improve blood-glucose control. Kale also contains a compound called alpha-lipoic acid, known to increase insulin sensitivity and prevent oxidative stress in people with diabetes. And, I'm happy to say, it tastes great and really fills you up because of the high fiber and protein content.

20. Salmon (Alaskan Wild Caught)

Salmon is notable for its exceptionally high level of omega-3 fatty acids. That translates into less inflammation, a better ratio of omega-6 to omega-3 fatty acids, improved cellular communication, increased cardiovascular health, better cognitive function, and improved metabolic markers. Even one four-ounce serving of salmon a week has measurable benefits for the heart, although two to three servings are recommended. Two eye conditions—macular degeneration and chronic dry eye—also profit from the consumption of salmon two to four times each week. Some interesting amino acids (they're called bioactive peptides) in salmon are being investigated for their positive effects on joint cartilage, insulin sensitivity, and inflammation of the intestinal lining. The most healthful salmon in terms of having less chemical and mercury contamination is Alaskan wild caught. Fortunately, this kind of salmon also rates high on the sustainability index, according to the Monterey Bay Aquarium Seafood Watch list. Be sure not to buy Atlantic salmon, a code name for far less healthful farmed salmon.

Ø Ø Ø

Some of these 20 Superfoods may be your Plus foods, while others may not. And in the process of Personalization, you might find other Plus foods as Mee McCormick did when she discovered that collard greens, kale, leafy greens, bok choy, cabbage, and brussels sprouts were particularly healing foods for her. There are tens of thousands of phytonutrients in plants alone, and we're just beginning to discover a few of their many properties.

Now that you're up to speed on nutritional science, the psychology of cravings, the importance of mindfulness, the art of Reboot and Personalization, and the role of Superfoods, let's take a look at your budget and see how you can eat a delicious PlantPlus Diet for less. After that, we'll get cookin'!

CHAPTER 26

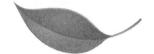

Eat Well for Less

*"The most remarkable thing about my mother is that
for thirty years she served the family nothing but leftovers.
The original meal has never been found."*

— CALVIN TRILLIN

Calvin Trillin's quote rings true for me. When I was a working mom with young kids, money was tight. It was all we could do to keep a roof over our heads and pay for child care, let alone spend a lot on food.

We grew a big organic garden and either froze or canned produce for winter. We picked apples with the kids in the fall and made giant batches of applesauce. We made pickles and picked berries for freezing and making jam, and we foraged for greens in the spring and for mushrooms (you gotta know what you're doing) in season. It was inexpensive family fun that we all remember with a lot of joy. I baked our own bread each week (the kids loved to help knead it), plus cookies and sourdough biscuits, and served lots of beans, rice, and pasta. If you can eat that many carbs, you're in luck, since those foods are relatively inexpensive.

But as you already know, at least for Gordon and me, such a high-carb diet didn't work well. When I tried it in my younger days, I couldn't keep any weight on, was constantly sick with bronchitis and pneumonia, had terrible migraines, and was always anxious. Although our diet was mostly whole foods and organic, it was simply unsuitable for my metabolism. The Plus foods that do suit my metabolic type are more expensive than beans, rice, and wheat. Dairy, fish, and poultry—particularly if you're committed to eating animal products from humanely raised, pasture-fed animals and wild-caught fish—is pricey. But we all have to budget according to priorities.

The Standard American Diet (SAD) is pricey, too. Processed food is cheap up-front, but eating it is like taking out a mortgage on your health with a balloon payment that suddenly comes due when poor health strikes.

Studies suggest that eating a whole-foods diet low in refined carbs—even if it's not a perfect match for you—is far healthier than relying on processed foods. Quinoa and brown rice, for example, are low on the glycemic index and high in fiber. If gluten-free whole grains are a Plus food for you, eating them is an inexpensive and delicious way to stretch your food dollar.

As mentioned earlier, my friend Mee Tracy McCormick, author of *My Kitchen Cure*, has created great recipes featuring these kinds of grains. She also cooks with beans. Soaking beans and grains before cooking to remove lectins and phytates improves their digestibility. They suit her metabolism well and form the backbone of the diet that keeps Mee's Crohn's disease (a chronic autoimmune condition) in check.

Known as the "Food Angel," Mee travels to rural churches and teaches congregants how to eat well for less. She can actually feed 50 people for $50. That's impressive. If she can do it, so can we. Where there's a will, there's always a way. Let's start with which foods to buy organic and what types of conventional produce are okay.

Organic vs. Conventional Produce

My prediction is that within 15 years, organic foods will be the norm, since in the long run they're cheaper to grow than crops reliant on weed killers and pesticides. But until that day comes, don't fret if your budget doesn't allow for a totally organic lifestyle. The most important foods to buy organic are foods containing fats like oil, butter, milk, cheese, and meat because most agricultural chemicals are fat soluble.

When it comes to fruits and veggies, the Environmental Working Group (EWG) writes: "The health benefits of a diet rich in fruits and vegetables outweigh the risks of pesticide exposure."[1] I agree. Eating conventionally grown produce is still better than eating no produce. But the fewer pesticides you eat, the better. So wash all produce as thoroughly as possible. I like to put it in a bowl of water, swish it around with my hands to get into all the little crevices, dump out the water, repeat a couple of times, and then spray the produce again with fresh water.

The EWG also publishes a useful list (updated annually) of the most heavily contaminated types of produce and the least contaminated. The *Dirty Dozen Plus* are worth buying organic—especially when you have children. You can save a little money on the *Clean Fifteen*, since they have relatively low pesticide levels. The EWG's "Shopper's Guide to Pesticides in Produce" for 2013, also available as a handy app for when you're shopping, is as follows:[2]

The Dirty Dozen Plus

Apples	Peaches
Celery	Potatoes
Cherry Tomatoes	Spinach
Cucumbers	Strawberries
Grapes	Sweet Bell Peppers
Hot Peppers	Kale and Collard Greens
Imported Nectarines	Summer Squash

The Clean Fifteen

Asparagus	Mangoes
Avocados	Mushrooms
Cabbage	Onions
Cantaloupe	Papayas
Sweet Corn	Pineapples
Eggplant	Frozen Sweet Peas
Grapefruit	Sweet Potatoes
Kiwi	

Eliminate Food Waste

Organic produce or any food is far less costly when you eat all that you buy. And both as individuals and as a nation, we waste a huge amount of food.

> According to the Natural Resources Defense Council (NRDC), $165 billion worth of food from homes, restaurants, and farms—approximately 40 percent of the food in the United States—goes uneaten every year and ends up in landfills. Its decomposition produces an unbelievable 16 percent of the methane that pollutes our environment. It's sobering to realize that people go hungry in the midst of such plenty. And think on this: *The average family of four loses $2,275 per year in food waste.*[3]

Wouldn't it be a better strategy to use that money to buy organic food and simply commit to throwing away less? There are even apps like *Green Egg Shopper* that alert you to use your food before it goes to waste. Most everyone buys produce that sits around in the fridge until it goes bad. How about using up those leftover green beans or half an onion in an omelet? How about taking five minutes (yes, it's that quick if you use my recipe) to bake those apples you bought on sale weeks ago?

Treat Leftovers Like Gold

In our house, leftovers are golden. They're beautiful food that's already prepared.

When you throw away leftovers that you've already cooked, you're wasting more than money. Out goes the food itself, plus the labor and resources it took to grow it, harvest it, ship it, store it, and sell it, the time it took you to prepare it, and the love that went into the cooking.

Here's an attitude adjustment for you:

> Leftovers aren't a booby prize that you're forced to eat; they're a reward for good cooking.

I love to make meals in the slow cooker or in my Dutch oven because the flavors mix and marry, creating rich and flavorful broths. When we're still enjoying them days later, it feels like we're at a restaurant. The shopping, cooking, and cleanup have already been done and we get to enjoy the goodies all over again.

We all have ways of saving money on food, and I'm happy to share a few that have worked for us.

A Few Money-Saving Tips

- Buy a food share from a local, organic Community Supported Agriculture (CSA) co-op. You're buying a share in the farm's crops, enabling them to survive and thrive. Our local CSA supplies vegetables, fruits, farm-made products, and free-range eggs. You can sometimes buy small, medium, or large shares and split the cost—and the bounty—with friends and neighbors.

- Stop the waste: Recycle, compost, and use the food that you buy rather than letting it go bad in your refrigerator. *It's helpful to reserve part of one shelf for leftovers and foods that need to be used soon.*

- If you're omnivorous, respect the life of the animal you're eating—and save money—by using every part of it. We freeze chicken and turkey carcasses, and the bones from any meat that we eat. These become the basis for stocks and soups.

- Shop twice a week, buying what's required for your weekly meal plan, and search the fridge for what you've got before you shop for more food. That way you eat fresh food and avoid waste.

- Limit restaurant meals. The food is often laced with bad oils, GMOs, pesticides, sugar, and refined carbs. Furthermore, it's expensive. Save both your health and your wallet by cooking at home.

- If you're omnivorous, use inexpensive cuts of meat in delicious soups and stews that last for several days. The cheaper cuts of beef—like flank, chuck, and blade—are actually the most flavorful. The lamb-stew recipe that you'll find in the next chapter, for instance, is made from a three-pound piece of relatively inexpensive shoulder roast. A $25 piece of meat sounds very expensive, but the pot of stew it makes provides 12 to 14 generous servings filled with vegetables and meat. Think about it. The per-portion cost is much cheaper than most fast-food meals.

Okay, 'nough said. As my friend Mee McCormick likes to say, "Let's get cookin'!"

CHAPTER 27

Joan and Gordon's Favorite PlantPlus Recipes

*"Cooking demands attention, patience,
and above all, a respect for the gifts of the earth.
It is a form of worship, a way of giving thanks."*

— JUDITH B. JONES

Good cooking is an art, a science, and a wonderful hobby. It grounds you back into the earth, your house, and your body—the most basic home that you'll ever have. The sweet, soft animal that it is (I thank poet Mary Oliver for that latter description), your body deserves appreciation, protection, and a little fun. In this chapter, I'll provide recipes for a long life and good living, all approved by Gordon, Chief Lab Rat and Food Critic for our in-home PlantPlus "Test Kitchen."

As you know, I'm not a chef. When home economics ended after fifth grade, so did my attendance at cooking classes. You might be a lot better at food preparation than I am. If that's the case, you'll be using, inventing, and modifying your own recipes sooner rather than later.

Mindful cooking encourages a spirit of curiosity and innovation: "Well, that dish was a sensational flop. So what did I learn?" Or "Wow, that dish was great! So what did I learn?"

Many of the omnivore recipes included here can be modified for vegans and vegetarians. I've developed most of them myself, but a few are Gordon's. Some are adapted from other sources as indicated, or were contributed by friends and colleagues.

You'll find a couple of recipes here for red meat—lamb and beef. The latest personalization experiment we're conducting is to eliminate almost all red meat from our diet to see if it affects total cholesterol particle number. Our cookbook (I keep a loose-leaf notebook of the recipes that we like) changes as we do, but if red meat is a Plus food for you, we hope you'll enjoy the two recipes I've included.

A Few Pointers

If you haven't spent much time in the kitchen lately, you might be a little bit rusty on common measurements. So before we start cooking, let's review some basic equivalents to help ensure that your cooking experiments turn out right. (And for cooks outside of the U.S., metric equivalent charts are included at the end of the book.)

3 teaspoons (tsp.) = 1 tablespoon (Tbsp.)
4 tablespoons = ¼ cup
1 cup = 8 fluid ounces or half a pint
2 cups = 1 pint
4 cups = 1 quart
4 quarts = 1 gallon
28 grams (g.) = 1 ounce (oz.)
454 grams = 1 pound (lb.)
16 ounces = 1 pound

Measuring Dry Ingredients

When a recipe calls for a tablespoon or less of a dry ingredient like a spice, baking soda, seeds, or flaxseed meal, get out your trusty measuring spoons and scoop up the ingredient so the appropriate spoon is completely full, then run the back of a knife over it to scrape off the excess. If a recipe calls for a heaping spoonful, don't scrape off the excess.

When measuring out quantities of a quarter cup or more, use your stainless-steel measuring cups in the same way you use the measuring spoons. Scoop up the ingredient, and remove the excess with the back of a knife. The same rules apply if you're measuring out coconut oil, which is a solid at room temperature.

Measuring Liquid Ingredients

When measuring one tablespoon or less of liquids, fill the measuring spoon up to the top. When measuring a quarter cup or more, use a glass measuring cup and hold it at eye level so that your measurement will be *exactly* on target. Even small variations can ruin some recipes like sauces, breads, cookies, and gelatin, which rely on chemical reactions. Soups, stews, and most main dishes are more forgiving, but it's wise to follow recipes as written—both here and elsewhere—at least once before you start making substitutions.

Tip: If you need to measure out an eighth of a cup, use a coffee scoop.

Measuring a Pound of Vegetables

Since the foundation of a PlantPlus lifestyle is a pound of vegetables a day, it's important to get a feeling for how much that is. Remember that 16 ounces equals one pound. In the spirit of making it easier to know what a pound of veggies looks like, I spent half an hour in the kitchen one day weighing all the vegetables in the house. It was fun as well as informative. If you've got kids, they'd make good assistants. Since hands-on learning works much better than blowing past words in a book, it's really helpful to do your own produce experiment.

Should you decide to try this, confine yourself to a single experiment. Once you've got a general idea of what a pound looks like, knock yourself out eating veggies, but don't go crazy calculating weights. Keep it simple. Life is complicated enough.

Greens

Tip: Prewashed salad greens (in a small clamshell container) = 5 ounces

Empty a package onto a large plate, and it will give you a point of reference for eyeballing a good amount of daily greens. Whether you use lettuce, kale, collards, chard, spinach, cilantro, parsley, or other greens, keep in mind what five ounces looks like. That's what to aim for. Of course, you might sometimes like to eat more. And inevitably, some days you'll eat less. But if you keep your eye on the prize, you'll be glad you did.

Remember the study from the *American Journal of Nutrition* conducted by a group of Israeli researchers. Their conclusion was that the macronutrient composition of the diet you eat is less important than how much of the diet consists of vegetables.[1] "Universal predictors of successful weight loss in the rapid weight loss phase across all diet strategies are increasing the weight of intake of vegetables and decreasing the weight of intake of sweets and cakes."[2]

So let's make it as easy as possible to increase the weight of veggies and decrease the weight of refined carbs in your diet.

Low-Starch Vegetables

Tip: 1 cup average = 4 ounces (cauliflower, broccoli, onions, cabbage, fennel, celery, radishes, green beans, and the like)

If you eat three cups of low-starch vegetables plus four to five cups of greens, you'll be right on target. That may sound like quite a bit, but when I chopped and weighed veggies for this chapter, I snacked on my experiment, polishing off a medium carrot (2 oz.), a big rib of celery (1½ oz.), and a quarter of a large red pepper (2 oz.). That was a third of a pound of veggies right there, gone effortlessly down the snack hatch.

Following the produce-weighing interlude, I roasted two cups of cauliflower, the rest of the red pepper, a cup of onion, a cup of green beans, and a few cashews for good measure. I ate almost two cups of that, plus some precooked shrimp for lunch. The veggies add up fast, if you keep the weight goal in mind. The magic of aiming for a pound a day is that this one new behavior—independent of anything else you do—creates mindfulness and focus.

Going hungry is a bad thing because it can lead to cheating and overeating. So when hunger strikes, choose a healthy snack. To paraphrase the poet Rumi, PlantPlus eating is "not a caravan of despair." Eating well is the final revenge of the diet wars.

Low-Glycemic Snack List

- ¼ cup nuts
- Two of my almond-flour cookies or a piece of almond-flour bread
- 3 or 4 roasted-sesame crackers or seed crackers with cheese, smoked salmon, hummus, roasted pepper, sliced turkey (not the slimy deli kind), or what have you
- An apple or most other fruits, with the exception of a ripe banana
- A hard-boiled egg
- A piece of cheese (you can carry prewrapped organic mozzarella sticks)

- A bag of cut vegetables

- SeaSnax brand seaweed sheets roasted in olive oil with a hint of sea salt. Half a package (2½ big square sheets) contains just 24 calories. As it says on the package, "Rip it up . . . Chomp it down!" Kids love it, too.

- After the Reboot, two or three cups of popcorn can work nicely for some people. Just make sure that it's nonGMO, as most corn in this country is genetically modified.

Streamlining Preparation

"Cooking is so popular today because it's the perfect mix of food and fun," says celebrity chef Emeril Lagasse. That's easy for him to say. It sure looks like fun when a chef empties those premeasured ingredients into the bowl with a flourish. That part takes only a few seconds. It's getting the ingredients ready in the first place that takes time.

Since you're likely to be your own sous chef unless a friend, spouse, or child pitches in, it pays to streamline the chopping. Cut up what you're likely to need for the next two or three days, and store it in glass containers in your refrigerator. Then, when it's time to cook or make a salad, you can pretend to be Emeril. I often pretend to be Julia Child, especially if I'm making onion soup, boning a duck, or dropping a fresh-roasted turkey on the floor. She sure had panache! The general principles for making your kitchen life simple are as follows:

- Plan your meals several days ahead of time so that you'll know what ingredients to buy.

- Wash and chop vegetables in advance.

- Create main dishes that will feed you and your household for more than one meal.

While washing dishes can be fun—at least according to Buddhist monk and mindfulness teacher Thich Nhat Hanh—life is simpler if you dirty as few dishes, pots, and pans as possible.

By putting aside a couple of hours twice a week as prep time, you can make a main-dish entrée that will last for several meals: Chop up veggies for salads, snacks, and quick dishes; bake; make desserts; bag snacks; and create staples like sauces and spice mixes.

Sample Breakfasts

Choose what you'd like, as there's no meal plan to follow. Just think about getting your veggies in, eating a few fermented things, and consuming enough protein to stay sated. You can choose from everything below:

- Yogurt smoothie
- Nondairy smoothie
- Sautéed greens
- Scrambled, poached, or fried eggs
- Veggie omelet
- Oatmeal for vegans, vegetarians, and some omnivores
- Almond-flour pancakes with blueberry sauce
- Almond-flour toast with nut butter and whole-fruit preserves
- Leftovers of any kind
- Sliced meat or cheese
- Smoked salmon or other fish
- A bowl of berries
- Half a grapefruit
- Breakfast on the run: a couple of hard-boiled eggs made in advance, a few nuts, and an apple

Sample Lunch Foods

- Giant salad with feta cheese or a few shavings of Parmesan; and tofu, tempeh, fish (canned sardines are good), poultry, or meat

- A serving of sauerkraut, kimchi, or pickled veggies to feed your microbiome

- Lettuce roll-ups with veggies, soy protein, fish, poultry, hummus, or meat

- Roasted vegetables

- Quesadillas made with chickpea tortillas

- Leftover main dishes

- Five- to ten-minute quickie meals like Turkey (or Tofu) Parmesan (recipe to follow)

- Whole fruit

- Cut-up veggies with salsa, hummus, or nut butter

- Baked apples

- One or two of Dr. J's (that's me) special cookies

- Almond bread

Sample Dinner Foods

- Savory entrées like soups, stews, and casseroles that are made ahead of time

- Salads

- Stir-fried vegetable medleys

- Roasted vegetables

- Mashed cauliflower or sweet potatoes

- Tofu, fish, poultry, or meat

- Almond loaf or focaccia bread

- Cut-up fruit or baked apples

- Gel-Yo (it looks like Jello, but it's delicious and very healthful—recipe to follow)

- Berries, apples, or nuts dipped in chocolate sauce

- Two squares of dark chocolate

Let's Start Cooking!

Savory Entrées

Our favorite protein-rich entrées are soups and stews. They last for several meals, getting better every day as the flavors mingle and marry. There's always something in the refrigerator, so quick meals are simple to rustle up. But some of the entrées I've included—like chicken piccata—are meals that you get to enjoy just once, since they need to be eaten fresh right out of the pan. If you're a vegetarian or a vegan, several of the entrées are suitable for you with just a few substitutions.

All entrées are grain-free and thus gluten-free.

LAMB STEW

Gordon and I both love lamb, although these days we're not eating it much since we're doing an experiment to see if the (near) elimination of red meat from our diet will lower total LDL particle number. In Chinese medicine, lamb is a tonic, and if you like the flavor, it makes a delicious and economical stew. While pasture-raised meat is more expensive than factory-farmed meat, lamb shoulder is an inexpensive, lean cut that goes a long way. The smell of this savory treat simmering in our big red enamel Dutch oven drives our standard poodles, Mitzi and Milo, wild. It makes us kind of crazy, too.

Serves 12–14

2–3 pounds of lamb shoulder, cut into one-inch cubes (you can substitute tempeh or poultry)

1 Tbsp. extra-virgin olive oil

2 Tbsp. or more to taste of Dr. J's Kickin' Spice Mix (see page 300)

1 32-oz. box of organic chicken, beef, or vegetable stock

1 6-oz. can of tomato paste

8 cups of vegetables, cut into chunks: 2 cups each of carrots, celery, onions, and fennel (use the stems as well as the bulb)

1 bunch of kale, sliced into strips through the ribs (see note below)

1 cup whole cranberries (fresh or frozen)

A dash of stevia

A note on cutting kale into ribbons: Hold several washed leaves together, with the stems pointing horizontally. Cut the leaves crosswise (right to left if you're right-handed, reversed for lefties) to create long strips with a section of rib in the center. Cut up all the stems, too.

Heat the olive oil in a large, heavy pot over medium heat. Brown the lamb, poultry, or tempeh in the oil; stir in the spices to coat; and then scoop the protein out of the pan. Add the stock and the tomato paste, stirring well to loosen any tasty tidbits on the bottom of the pan. Then add the protein back in; and put in the vegetables and kale, cranberries, and stevia. Simmer at very low heat for 90 minutes to two hours, until the meat is tender. Keep tasting the stew, adding more spice mix (or not) as needed. The vegan alternative takes only about an hour. It's done when the vegetables are fork tender.

This stew is great by itself, served over spaghetti squash, or accompanied by a slice of toasted almond bread to dip in the savory gravy. Add a big salad, some roasted cauliflower or asparagus, and you're good to go.

Omnivore variation: Use beef chuck instead of lamb.

Spice lovers: Add two diced jalapeño peppers. Delicious and not too hot.

THAI SHRIMP-AND-SCALLOP CURRY

We all need a few tasty and festive company dishes. This delicate but hearty dish features the tastes of Thailand—coconut, cilantro, chili, and piquant fish sauce with shrimp and scallops. I've simplified the recipe, which has many variations, and taken my final inspiration from a *Bon Appétit* recipe that I found on the Internet. Gordon's favorite cookbook, by the way, is *Bon Appétit's Fast, Easy, Fresh.* Many of the recipes are wonderful as is, or easily adaptable to a PlantPlus lifestyle. This dish can be reheated, and it can last for two to three days.

Serves 8

1 pound large shrimp, peeled and deveined
1 pound bay scallops, washed and carefully dried
2 Tbsp. coconut oil
1 bunch scallions (sliced thin, keeping the white and green parts separate)
3 cloves garlic (minced or pressed)
½ cup chopped cilantro
2 Tbsp. red curry paste (or 6 Tbsp. green)
½ tsp. chili powder
1 can (about 14 oz.) light, unsweetened coconut milk
2 tsp. fish sauce
1½ cups of water
2 large carrots sliced into thin rounds
4 cups thinly sliced bok choy
¼ cup chopped basil

Heat the coconut oil in a large saucepan or Dutch oven over medium heat. Add the white parts of the scallions, the garlic, and a heaping tablespoon of cilantro. Sauté for a couple of minutes until fragrant, being careful not to burn the garlic. Stir in the curry paste and chili powder; then add the coconut milk, fish sauce, and water. When that's simmering nicely, add the carrots and cover the pot. Let it cook for about five minutes, and then layer the bok choy, shrimp, and scallops on top. The seafood will cook quickly, in about five minutes. You'll know when the scallops are done because they lose their translucency and become opaque. The shrimp will turn pink and curl up. Stir everything together and sprinkle the curry lightly with the rest of the cilantro, chopped basil, and the green parts of the scallions before serving. (You may want to save some of the chopped toppings for leftovers.)

KITCHEN SINK CHICKEN OR TURKEY SOUP

We love this soup so much that it's on the menu every few weeks. I call it Kitchen Sink Chicken Soup because it's usually based on whatever chicken, turkey, or duck leftovers are lurking in the freezer, plus any vegetables other than broccoli, cauliflower, or brussels sprouts that need to be used up. Sometimes I've got a few frozen turkey legs, a turkey carcass (what a prize!), some turkey meat, or a chicken carcass. The bones add a lot of flavor, and I agree with proponents of ancestral diets that bone broths are good for you. You can use the following recipe as a guide in case you don't have any leftovers for the soup. Improvisation is the spice of life, so go to town with what you've got.

Serves 8–10

1 whole chicken, cut into quarters
1 Tbsp. olive oil
1 very large onion or two medium onions, cut into chunks
1 red bell pepper, cut into ½-inch pieces
1 bunch of curly kale, kale ribs, or collards, sliced in ribbons (see the note on page 264 about slicing kale into ribbons)
6 ribs of celery, cut into chunks
6 medium carrots, cut into rounds
1 large can of San Marzano Italian tomatoes (cut each tomato into fourths)
1 tsp. ground ginger

2 tsp. turmeric

2 32-oz. cartons of chicken stock

1 Tbsp. herbes de Provence

Salt and pepper to taste

Heat a tablespoon of olive oil in a big, heavy soup pot over medium heat. Swirl it around to cover the bottom of the pot, and add the chicken—skin and all. Sauté it lightly on both sides and remove. Add the vegetables, sautéing them until the onions and greens start to wilt, and then add the ginger and turmeric and stir it all up. Put the chicken back in; and add the stock, the herbes de Provence, and perhaps a teaspoon of salt and pepper. Simmer on low heat, and after about an hour, taste the soup, and adjust the seasonings and add more stock if needed. Take out the chicken, which should be falling off the bone, and hunt around for any stray bones in the pot. Once the chicken cools, pull the meat off the bones, and add it to the soup. Any fat will float to the top of the soup and congeal in the fridge. You can skim it off with ease.

Ancestral eaters prize chicken fat for cooking, as did my mom, who called it *schmaltz*. It pays to be mindful while eating the soup, since there may be a bone or two hiding in the bounty.

MISO-GLAZED TOFU OR TEMPEH (COMPLIMENTS OF MARILYN TAM)

Marilyn is an excellent chef, and it's always a treat to eat at her home. She can make tempeh sing, and for me, that's no easy task!

Serves 3–6

6 pieces tofu or tempeh, cut into fillet-sized servings

½ cup light-yellow miso

5 tsp. rice vinegar

2 Tbsp. soy sauce

¼ tsp. cayenne pepper

¼ cup olive oil

Toasted sesame seeds and chopped chives for garnish

Preheat the broiler. Blend the miso, rice vinegar, soy sauce, and cayenne pepper in a blender. Add the olive oil, and blend until smooth. Pour half the mixture over the tofu or tempeh.

Broil the tofu/tempeh eight inches from the broiler until it begins to brown (approximately three minutes). Then bake it at 450 degrees until warm in the center (approximately an additional five minutes).

Drizzle the remaining miso mixture over the tofu/tempeh, if desired, and garnish with sesame seeds and chives. Serve with green vegetables, such as sautéed broccoli or spinach.

EGGPLANT PARMESAN

This is Gordon's favorite meal. It takes a little time to make this dish (about 30 minutes), but it's well worth the effort. It's a bit like vegetable lasagna, except there's no lasagna—rounds of eggplant take its place. While we prepare this with a traditional ricotta-cheese filling and bubbly mozzarella on top, vegans can blend up silken tofu with Italian herbs and substitute that for the easy, cheesy filling. There's only the two of us, but we're happy to eat this for as long as it lasts.

Serves 9

1 large eggplant cut in ¾-inch rounds, skin left on
¼ tsp. salt
¼ tsp. fresh ground pepper
1 egg
1 8-oz. container ricotta cheese
2 tsp. Italian herbs
1 medium onion, diced
1 red or green bell pepper, diced
2 cloves garlic
1 bunch of kale, sliced in ribbons (see page 264 for instructions)
6 oz. fresh white mushrooms, sliced thin

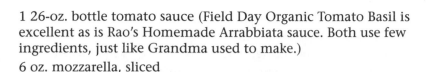
1 26-oz. bottle tomato sauce (Field Day Organic Tomato Basil is excellent as is Rao's Homemade Arrabbiata sauce. Both use few ingredients, just like Grandma used to make.)

6 oz. mozzarella, sliced

Preheat the oven to 375 degrees. Spray a cookie sheet liberally with olive oil, lay the eggplant rounds down on the sheet, and season with salt and pepper. Spray with more olive oil. (Use a Misto sprayer; it's a lot cheaper than buying spray cans, and you get to control the quality of the oil.) Bake the eggplant for 20 minutes. In the meantime, do the other prep.

To make the filling, beat the egg in a bowl and stir in the ricotta cheese and Italian herbs. For the vegan version, beat tofu in a bowl with Ener-G Egg Replacer (follow package directions for amount).

Sauté the onions, peppers, and garlic in a spray of olive oil; and then add the kale and mushrooms. When the vegetables are wilted, take off the heat.

Using a 9" by 13" glass casserole dish, pour enough of the marinara sauce into the bottom of the dish to cover it easily. Layer the roasted eggplant on top of the sauce. Next add a layer of veggies, the ricotta or tofu filling, another layer of sauce, and then top with the sliced mozzarella. Cover the dish with aluminum foil, and bake for 30 minutes. Take the foil off, and bake for an additional 30 minutes. Let cool for 15 minutes before digging in.

Tip: If you use a microwave (some people don't, but we do), you can easily warm leftovers. Take a piece, top it with a fresh slice of mozzarella, and nuke it for two minutes. It's a feast!

BRISKET IN ONION SAUCE

I'm always on the lookout for ways to incorporate onions into our meals since they're a potent prebiotic. Although pasture-raised meat is more expensive than factory-farmed meat, it's still economical when you choose cuts like chuck roast and brisket. These are among the most flavorful cuts of beef—they're moist and tender when slow cooked. This is my mother Lilly's brisket recipe (more or less). I make this on Jewish holidays, so it's a rare treat. Like most cooks of her day, my mom threw in a little of this and a little of that. I remember her old cookbook from the Temple Sisterhood. It had units of measurement like "Use a piece of butter the size of an egg." Now you know why I'm used to improvising.

Serves 8–12

3-pound piece grass-fed brisket with fat trimmed off
1 Tbsp. olive oil
4 very large onions
1 Tbsp. turmeric
1 Tbsp. cumin
Salt and pepper to taste
1 20-oz. can plum tomatoes (cut the tomatoes into quarters)
½ cup organic, sugar-free ketchup
2 Tbsp. Worcestershire sauce
8 carrots, cut into one-inch chunks

Fire up a big, enamel Dutch oven or soup pot on medium heat, and brown the brisket in a tablespoon of olive oil. While the meat is browning, which will take about five minutes on each side, cut the onions into rings. Take out the brisket and lay it aside.

Brown the onions in the same pot, adding a little water if they start to stick. Stir frequently, and don't let them burn, which makes onions bitter. When they start to caramelize (turning soft and brown), add the turmeric, cumin, salt, and pepper; and stir well. Then stir in the tomatoes, ketchup, Worcestershire, and carrots. Return the brisket to the pot, and cover with the onion sauce.

Let the brisket simmer on very low heat for about three hours, turning occasionally and stirring the sauce. The brisket will shrink quite a bit as it cooks, but the key to eating meat (if you do) is to keep the portions small. Three to four ounces max is best. Meat is ideally more of a condiment than a main course. This dish goes well with a big kale salad.

CHICKEN OR FISH PICCATA

This recipe is a superstreamlined version of an old favorite. The secret to great flavor if you're panfrying fish or chicken is to use a half-butter, half–olive oil mixture. It makes a delicious difference. Pan- or oven-fried foods are usually dipped in flour, egg, and bread crumbs; however, in this simple recipe, you just press the chicken or fish into almond flour seasoned with salt and pepper.

Serves 4

1 lb. flounder or sole* fillets or 1 lb. chicken breasts cut lengthwise through the middle to yield 4 thin fillets
1 cup almond flour
¼ tsp. salt (optional)
¼ tsp. pepper
2 Tbsp. butter
2 Tbsp. olive oil
2 Tbsp. capers, drained and rinsed
½ cup white wine or chicken stock
Juice of two lemons (about ⅓ cup)
¼ cup chopped parsley

In a shallow dish or bowl, mix the almond flour and salt and pepper; then dredge the fillets in the seasoned flour and lightly shake off any excess. Heat a large frying pan over medium heat. Put in 1 Tbsp. butter and 1 Tbsp. olive oil, and mix to cover the bottom of the pan. Your fillets should sizzle when you put them in; if not, the heat is too low. Fry fish for about three minutes per side. Chicken will take about five minutes per side. Remove the fillets when they're cooked through, and put them aside.

Preparing the sauce: Add the remaining butter and olive oil to the pan, and then add the capers. Smash them up a bit with the back of a spoon to release their briny flavor. Pour in the white wine or chicken stock, and scrape the bottom of the pan to release all the little bits of savory goodness. Cook the sauce down for about two minutes to thicken it. Stir in the lemon juice and the parsley; then return the fillets to the pan and spoon the sauce over them. Heat them through for a minute or two, and serve right away.

*According to the Monterey Bay Seafood Watch list, sole and flounder are good choices in terms of sustainability and safety. If you go to www.seafoodwatch.org/cr/cr_seafoodwatch/download .aspx, and click on your region of the country, you can download a list of best choices, good alternatives, and fish and shellfish to avoid. Print it out, and take it with you when you shop.

ORIENTAL LETTUCE WRAPS

These take a little time to prepare, but the filling lasts in the fridge for a few days so that one preparation can provide a gourmet treat for a couple of meals. These also make wonderful appetizers and are easy to serve since they can be prepared ahead of time and reheated just before serving.

Serves 10–12

½ lb. shredded, cooked chicken breast; or ½ lb. minced, cooked shrimp; or ½ lb. diced tempeh
2 Tbsp. olive oil
½ inch gingerroot, peeled and minced
2 cloves garlic minced
6 scallons thinly sliced (white and green parts)
1 cup diced red peppers
½ cup shredded carrots
2 cups thin-sliced bok choy
2 Tbsp. gluten-free soy sauce
2 Tbsp. mirin (rice-wine vinegar)
1 Tbsp. hoisin sauce
1 tsp. sriracha hot sauce
½ cup coarsely chopped raw cashews
1 head iceberg lettuce cut in half, leaves washed and spun dry; or
2 romaine hearts separated into single leaves (at least 12 leaves)

Heat the olive oil in a big frying pan on medium high. Add the minced ginger and garlic, stirring for a few seconds. Then add the vegetables. Stir-fry for two to three minutes, until the vegetables start to wilt. *Do not overcook.* Add the chicken (or shrimp or tempeh), and stir. Add the soy sauce, mirin, hoisin sauce, and sriracha; stir for another minute or two. Turn out immediately onto a serving platter. Serve with the lettuce, wrapping a few tablespoons of the filling in each lettuce leaf and topping with chopped cashews.

Salads and Vegetables

KALE SALAD

I snubbed my nose at kale for years and never thought that this sturdy, tough leaf would make a good salad . . . but now I'm more than happy to eat my words. This is fun to make and completely, unexpectedly, outrageously delicious. It lasts up to three days in the refrigerator.

Serves 6–8

1 large bunch noncurly kale, ribs removed, leaves cut into ½-inch slices
3 Tbsp. olive oil
¼ tsp. salt
¼ tsp. pepper
2 Tbsp. white balsamic vinegar or raw apple-cider vinegar
1 large fennel bulb sliced thin and cut into small pieces
1 Granny Smith or Honeycrisp apple, diced
4 big, red or purple radishes, diced
½ cup raw or toasted sunflower seeds

Note: Cut the kale leaves off the ribs, and save the ribs to use in soups and stews.

Put the cut-up kale leaves in a bowl, and pour the olive oil over them. With clean hands, massage the oil into the kale, squeezing it between your fingers to break down the tough fibers. (A very sensuous deed that's not optional—it makes the dish.) Add the salt and pepper, vinegar, fennel, apples, and radishes; and mix it all together earnestly with your hands. Sprinkle with sunflower seeds before serving.

BEAN-SPROUT SALAD

This is one of my favorite salads ever. You can either buy mung bean sprouts or sprout them yourself. We just ordered a sprouting kit from Amazon to make our kitchen into a garden. It takes just a few days to make a batch of sprouts.

Serves 2–4

8 oz. mung bean sprouts
⅓ cup scallions sliced thin (white and green parts)
1 Tbsp. toasted sesame seeds

Mix the sprouts, scallions, and toasted sesame seeds with the dressing. For the dressing, shake up the following in a jar with a lid:

1 Tbsp. olive oil
1 Tbsp. toasted sesame oil
2 Tbsp. mirin (rice-wine vinegar)
1 clove garlic minced

This salad lasts for up to two days in the refrigerator and gets better as it marinates.

BROCCOLI SLAW

I got inspired by my colleague Josh, the King of Slaws, whom you met earlier, to make this simple, delicious, nutritious cruciferous wonder.

Serves 4

8-oz. bag organic broccoli slaw
¼ cup apple-cider vinegar (I use Bragg's organic, raw, unfiltered.)
1 Tbsp. gluten-free tamari
1 tsp. Truvia or equivalent in stevia (optional)
½ tsp. Dr. J's Kickin' Spice Mix (see page 300)
2 Tbsp. sunflower seeds

Mix all ingredients together. This slaw could probably last for two to three days in the fridge, but Gordon and I always finish it by the second day. It gets more flavorful as it sits and marinates.

MIXED-GREEN SALAD WITH PECANS AND GOAT-FETA CHEESE

This delicious salad is a one-dish meal. We top it with a slice of goat-feta cheese. We took that inspiration from the fresh, satisfying salads we enjoyed one summer while touring the Greek islands.

Serves 2

2 cups arugula
2 cups mixed greens or chopped romaine lettuce
1 cup thinly sliced fennel
2 large radishes, chopped
1 avocado, sliced
1–2 scallions, sliced thin
½ cup toasted pecans (recipe follows)
2 slices goat-feta cheese

Combine the first six ingredients in a large bowl, and dress with Gordon's Vinaigrette (see page 303). Divide the salad into two dishes, and top each with toasted pecans and a slice of goat-feta cheese.

To toast the pecans:

2 cups pecans
2 Tbsp. maple syrup

Combine the pecans and maple syrup in a bowl, and mix well. Add to a heated cast-iron frying pan, and stir on medium heat until the nuts are toasted. A little bit of maple syrup in a recipe like this won't break the carb bank, but it sure adds a lot of flavor. Use a half cup of the toasted pecans for the mixed-green salad. The remaining nuts make a perfect snack!

POACHED GREEN BEANS

Serves 2–4

1 lb. green beans
Water to cover

Wash the green beans, cut off the ends, and either leave them whole or cut them into pieces as you wish. Put the beans in a cast-iron frying pan with water to just barely cover them, and cook at medium-high heat for five to ten minutes until al dente (crisp tender). These are so delicious if you don't overcook them.

THE BEST ROASTED CAULIFLOWER

This recipe—compliments of Marilyn Tam—is fast, simple, and simply delicious! You can do the same thing with brussels sprouts or a combination of the two. These veggies are yummy and are an aesthetically pleasing treat if you combine vegetables of different colors. I ate this at Marilyn's house and was amazed how much better these roasted veggies were than any others I'd ever had. The high heat is what does the trick. Marilyn uses a 500-degree oven, and I generally roast veggies at 450.

Serves 4–6

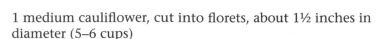

1 medium cauliflower, cut into florets, about 1½ inches in diameter (5–6 cups)

¼ cup extra-virgin olive oil

1 Tbsp. minced garlic (If you love garlic, use more as Marilyn does.)

2 Tbsp. lemon juice

½ tsp. sea salt or to taste

½ tsp. black pepper or a sprinkling of cayenne pepper

Chopped chives or parsley, for garnish

Preheat the oven to 450 degrees. Place the cauliflower florets in a large glass pan or roasting pan. Drizzle the olive oil over the cauliflower, and season with the garlic, lemon juice, salt, and pepper. Mix well. Bake for 15 minutes, stirring occasionally to ensure even roasting. Remove from the oven, and garnish with chopped chives or parsley. Serve immediately, or add to green salads. Delicious! (For added protein or to serve as a main dish, cube some tempeh and toss it in with the cauliflower before roasting.)

MEE TRACY McCORMICK'S CLASSIC CAESAR SALAD

By now, you're familiar with my friend Mee, who is a beautiful lady, inside and out. As I mentioned earlier, folks know her as the Kitchen Angel because she shares her whole-foods cooking gifts and has helped so many people with gut problems get well. Mee let me lift this recipe lock, stock, and barrel from her book, *My Kitchen Cure*.

Serves 4

1 head romaine lettuce

1 cup gluten-free croutons (optional)

½ cup Mee's Caesar Dressing (recipe follows)

1 avocado, sliced

4 lemon slices

Slice romaine head lengthwise in quarters. Remove base and chop lettuce into one-inch pieces. Place in a mixing bowl, and toss with croutons and Mee's Caesar Dressing. Arrange avocado slices on individual plates or in a serving bowl, and garnish with lemon slices. You could also serve with tempeh, organic chicken, or fish.

MEE'S CAESAR DRESSING

Makes 2 cups

1 cup olive oil
¾ cup water
¼ cup miso
¼ cup lemon juice
2 garlic cloves, chopped
1 Tbsp. capers
¾ tsp. sea salt
¼ tsp. black pepper
⅛ tsp. white pepper

Puree all ingredients in a blender. Store in a glass jar up to four days in the refrigerator.

GORDON'S SHIITAKE VEGGIES

Mushrooms are good food, and shiitake mushrooms are particularly popular at our house. Gordon likes to cut up some shiitakes and marinate them in gluten-free tamari.

Serves 4–6

½ lb. shiitake mushrooms, quartered
1 tsp. gluten-free tamari
1 Tbsp. mirin (rice wine)
1 Tbsp. extra-virgin olive oil
1 tsp. finely chopped ginger
½ pound green beans, cut into 1½-inch lengths

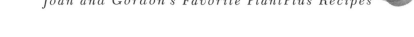

½ large red pepper, diced
1 Tbsp. pan-toasted sesame seeds
1 tsp. toasted sesame oil (optional)

Mix the shiitakes with the tamari, mirin, olive oil, and ginger; and allow to marinate for at least 20 minutes. Add a spray of olive oil in a large skillet over medium heat; and then stir-fry the green beans, red pepper, and marinated shiitakes until tender-crisp. Sprinkle with toasted sesame seeds or toasted sesame oil, if desired. You can add any kind of protein to this dish.

Simple Five- to Ten-Minute Meals

LUNCH OR DINNER SALADS

Salads make great quick meals, and you can easily eat four or five cups of greens in a serving. I used to make salads in bowls, but the bowls we have are too small for the giant salads that are such a big part of the PlantPlus lifestyle. While we generally use salad plates for our main dishes, we now use dinner plates for our salads. How's that for being contrary? If you eat a salad for lunch three or four days a week, you'll keep your digestive system well toned and humming along unless you're suffering from IBS or Crohn's disease and have a stomach lining that needs to heal before it can rejoice with too many uncooked greens.

Load up your plate with any kind of greens you choose—four to five cups. It's always nice to include some spicy ones, such as arugula. Fortunately, you can buy a variety of prewashed greens in five-ounce containers, which makes them superportable. Cut half an avocado into chunks; and add some slices of red pepper, apples, radishes, or whatever you've got that's prechopped and ready to go. Toss in a few cashews, almonds, or sunflower seeds for crunch. Add some cubed feta, cooked chicken or shrimp, sardines, or Marilyn's miso-glazed tofu or tempeh. Dress the salad with a light, bright vinaigrette, and you've got a feast.

HOT CHICKEN ON THE FLY

On busy nights when we've run out of precooked entrées, Gordon and I sometimes pick up an organic, free-range rotisserie chicken for dinner. We pair it with a roasted sweet potato—half for each of us and the skins for the poodles—and make a big salad with prechopped ingredients from the fridge. (Keep in mind that unless you're a vegetarian, tubers aren't on the Reboot menu.) The leftover chicken is great for lunch salads, and the carcass goes into the freezer to use in soup.

TURKEY (OR TOFU) PARMESAN QUICKIE

I love Italian food but don't miss the pasta. This quick lunch is ready to go in ten minutes.

Serves 1

3–4 oz. ground-turkey patty (we keep them in the freezer) or
4 oz. tofu
2 cups leftover kale or other cooked veggies
½ cup good-quality bottled tomato sauce (or your own if you've got some on hand)
1 oz. slice mozzarella cheese (optional)

Sauté the turkey patty or tofu in a spray of olive oil. Surround with the kale or other cooked veggies, top with tomato sauce and mozzarella, and cover the pan. In a few minutes, it will be heated through, and the mozzarella (if you use it) will be melted—stringy and delicious. Voilà. You've got a big, yummy, filling lunch.

SIMPLE LETTUCE WRAPS

You can make a simple wrap out of any protein by taking an ounce or two of the protein and combining it with lettuce, tomatoes, cucumbers, roasted vegetables, sprouts, cheese, hummus, or whatever PlantPlus foods you like. Use good-quality, organic mayonnaise, mustard, Vegenaise, or hot sauce to spice it up.

Fermented Stuff

Fermented vegetables are a staple in many cultures. My former mother-in-law, who came from Ukraine, always made delicious pickles and sauerkraut. She used big crocks covered with plates and weighed down with stones.

I didn't relish the thought (pardon the pun) of making vats of smelly stuff in the kitchen, but a friend told me that she made pickles frequently in quart jars on her countertop with no fuss, smell, or bother. She used a simple system called the Perfect Pickler (www.perfectpickler.com). I have no business deal with these pickling mavens other than having purchased their efficient little fermenting setup: a jar top with a hole in the center and a rubber gasket that fits any size wide-mouth canning jar; a plastic valve that fits in the hole and keeps out mold; and a great booklet that ushers you into the world of fermentation and provides 25 recipes.

Since cucumbers were out of season when our kit arrived, we started our culinary adventure with sauerkraut. Why not buy it at the store, you ask? Well, the good stuff in the refrigerator case that hasn't been pasteurized costs a fortune—about $8 for a small bottle. Too expensive for us. Furthermore, we thought that pickling might be a fun adventure. And it really is.

If you're wondering whether it's safe, the answer, generally speaking, is yes—unless you blow yourself up making root beer or other fermented beverages. And you won't be dining on botulinum toxin if you follow the simple instructions. Prior to trying our hand at this simple art, we read *The Art of Fermentation* by Sandor Ellix Katz. The Foreword to this veritable bible of pickling—which covers the art, science, and deep enjoyment of the craft—was written by Michael Pollan, one of my most esteemed food heroes.

Sauerkraut is a bit more labor intensive than pickled veggies, because after you chop up the cabbage, you have to massage salt into it and let it sit until it forms a brine. Then you pour it into jars. But the 20 minutes or so that we invested in making our own kraut paid off handsomely. One head of cabbage makes one quart and one pint of outstanding sauerkraut.

If you want to see what the pickling process looks like and how you can get started in just a few minutes, watch the short video on the homepage of www.perfectpickler.com.

Smoothies

DR. J'S PROBIOTIC, ANTI-INFLAMMATORY, SUPER-DELICIOUS, BERRY-YOGURT SMOOTHIES

It took me a year to find a delicious smoothie that wasn't so full of fruits high in the glycemic index that they spiked my blood sugar and left me weak with hunger an hour later. This super-antioxidant smoothie is so good that I crave it—and I'm very hard to please. It makes a good breakfast by itself, or a great addition to other foods, and it keeps me full until lunch. The fruit variations are almost endless, so we change them up depending on the berries and other low-glycemic fruits that are available.

Serves 1–2

1 cup plain, unsweetened organic yogurt (cow, goat, or soy)
½ cup frozen organic cranberries
1 cup organic mixed berries (We buy the frozen organic blueberry, strawberry, and blackberry mix from Costco.)
1 small apple
1 inch gingerroot
1 inch turmeric root
½ tsp. cinnamon
1 Tbsp. Truvia or equivalent in stevia (since cranberries are sour)
4–6 ice cubes (if using fresh fruit rather than frozen)
Water—enough to come up to the top of the other ingredients

I'm fortunate to have a Vitamix, which is so powerful that there's no need to either peel or chop the ginger or turmeric first. If you're using another kind of blender, peel the roots and chop them into smaller pieces. Place all the ingredients into the blender and process first at low speed, scraping the sides of the container if necessary. Finish processing at high speed.

We like our smoothies gingery and spicy, bright and exciting, but you can add less ginger if it suits you. Any kind of berries work well in this smoothie. We've particularly enjoyed this with organic cherries, either mixed with blueberries or by themselves. You could add a pear instead of an apple or make peach or apricot smoothies. Costco sells several different organic frozen fruits, including cherries, at a very reasonable price. If you're using fresh berries, add four to six ice cubes before blending to chill the smoothie.

BLUEBERRY-LAVENDER SMOOTHIE
(COMPLIMENTS OF MEE TRACY McCORMICK)

Here's what Mee says about this tasty smoothie:

When I was pregnant with both of my babies, I was addicted to lavender. Once I discovered this smoothie, I was hooked! In addition, it's packed full of cancer fighters and inflammation reducers—bring on those blueberries, baby! Toss in the antioxidant-, mineral-, and vitamin-rich spinach to get that extra kick in nutritional value and the lavender to aid in calming and soothing the body. It's the perfect treat to kick back and relax, and kids love it, too!

Serves 2–4

5 cups organic blueberries, fresh or frozen
2 cups almond milk
1 handful of spinach
1 Tbsp. brown-rice syrup
1 Tbsp. dried lavender
1 tsp. vanilla
Pinch of salt

Add all the ingredients in the blender, and whiz it up.

DAIRY-FREE POWER SMOOTHIE

Marilyn Tam came to stay with us for a few days when I was helping her brainstorm for one of her excellent books, *The Happiness Choice*. She arrived with a few supplies to make her morning smoothie, which she sometimes drinks throughout the afternoon. I watched her fill the Vitamix with an astonishing array of stuff. As the blender revved up, she smiled. "Ah," she purred, "the sound of health." Here's how the master makes a smoothie:

What follows are the basic things for a delicious and nutritious smoothie, which will power you up! This is a general recipe for you to experiment with so that you can customize yours based on your taste and the availability of fresh fruits and vegetables. That's the key—choose what's freshest and organic whenever you can. Chop up everything to a reasonable size (two inches, approximately). If you are using a standard blender, you may have to experiment to see how much you can make at a time. You will be amazed how powerful even a regular blender is. Of course, I love my Vitamix; I use it daily for making smoothies, soups, hummus, and more. (I do not own their stock or have any affiliation with them at all.)

Start with three kinds of fruit—you can have more if you wish, and it's good to vary them because every fruit has a different nutritional profile. I've noted which ones *ideally have to be organic* based on the pesticides used on the particular fruit or vegetable (generally, if at all possible, use only organic). If you're pressed for time, there are several kinds of frozen fruits and vegetables that you can use—some of them are even organic.

Fruits

Use three kinds of fruits:
Lemon (use only half)
Oranges
Apples (only organic)
Bananas

Papaya
Pears (only organic)
Peaches (only organic)
Nectarines (only organic)
Grapes (only organic)
Strawberries (only organic)
Blueberries
Raspberries
Kiwis
Avocado (use half, depending on size)
Coconut oil (only organic; use 2 tablespoons per blenderful)

Vegetables

Use two or more kinds of vegetables:
Carrots
Zucchini (only organic)
Celery (only organic; strong tasting, use small amount)
Tomato
Kale (only organic; strong tasting, use small amount)
Collard greens (rather strong tasting)
Spinach
Beets (strong tasting, use small amount)
Ginger (Start with a small amount as it can get a bit spicy. Ginger is very good for digestion, intestinal support, and reducing inflammation.)

Raw Nuts and Seeds

Sunflower seeds, pumpkin seeds, almonds, cashews, and so on: Use two handfuls per large blenderful (eight-cup capacity blender). If possible, soak the nuts from 20 minutes to two hours, or even overnight, and rinse and discard the water before you use. This reduces the tannins in the nuts, increases the enzymatic activity to help digestibility, and starts the sprouting process to enhance the nutritional profile. You can keep soaked nuts in the refrigerator—just be sure to rinse before use.

Optional Goodies

Greens powder: There are many kinds on the market. Experiment with different ones—and read the labels, as there are some with vegetable protein included, which you may want to factor in if you also add nuts to your smoothie. Greens powders all taste different, so see what tastes good and is good for you.

Chia seeds: Available from most health-food stores; use one tablespoon or more per blenderful.

Chlorella or spirulina: Available from most health-food stores; look at the info on the packaging and add enough for two servings per Vitamix blenderful or one serving per regular blenderful. Chlorella and spirulina can be strong tasting, so take it easy at first.

Liquid minerals/fulvic mineral complex: Available from good health-food stores; sometimes this is combined in a liquid-vitamins mix (see label for amount).

Directions

The ratio of fruits to vegetables is dependent on your taste, so if you're somewhat new at this, use twice as much, or more, fruit than vegetables—especially if you're including strong-tasting ones like kale, celery, or spinach.

Fill the blender with your selected items, add filtered water—fill only to the bottom of the top layer of chopped-up ingredients—and blend. Add more water as needed, and blend till smooth. Pour and enjoy!

There you have it! Smoothies are delicious *and* nutritious, and they're wonderful for breakfast or an afternoon snack. Make one for yourself the night before so that you're ready to go in the morning. Just blend it again, and breakfast is served!

Baked Goods

GRAIN-FREE TORTILLAS

You can make great wraps in lettuce leaves, but from time to time you might hanker for a doughy little wrap. If beans are a Plus food for you, you're going to love these low-carb, high-fiber tortillas. They're essentially sturdy crepes. While traditional chickpea flatbreads are made of only three ingredients—chickpea flour, water, and olive oil—I've invented a recipe for thin, but sturdy, chickpea tortillas.

Serves 2–4

1 egg
¼ cup chickpea (garbanzo bean) flour
¼ cup soy, rice, or almond milk
About 2 Tbsp. water
Seasonings of your choice

In a mixing bowl, beat the egg and mix in the chickpea flour and your favorite nondairy milk. The batter needs to be the consistency of heavy cream, so you might have to add a tablespoon or two of water. After making this a couple of times, you'll get the hang of the desired consistency. For added flavor, I prefer a little oregano, salt, and pepper; but you can use the seasonings of your choice.

Spray some olive oil on a hot cast-iron griddle, pour on the batter, and spread it out with the back of a ladle. It will bubble like a pancake. Flip when it's set, and cook it for a minute on the other side. *Yes!* I made a grilled-cheese quesadilla for lunch—complete with slices of tasty dill pickles inside—with the very first one of these ever to come off our griddle. Tomatoes and other veggies are great in these, too.

GOLDEN ALMOND BREAD

The Internet is awash in recipes for bread made out of various gluten-free grains; however, that kind of bread is bursting with high-glycemic carbs and not appropriate for a PlantPlus Diet. So I zeroed in on making home-baked goods with almond flour and flaxseed meal—both of which are very low in carbs and high in nutrients and flavor.

I've baked at least a dozen types of almond-flour bread (I use finely ground, plain old blanched almonds). I finally settled on a recipe from Jorge Cruise that I adapted by adding flaxseed meal for extra nutrition and spices to step up the flavor. It's the simplest and most delicious of all the breads I've made. It has a moist texture, a savory flavor, and a magnificent golden color because of the turmeric. The loaf slices beautifully and makes good toast. Before I discovered this bread, I had put the toaster away in the pantry. Now it has come back out again.

There are three cups of almond flour in the loaf, so if you cut it into 12 slices, each will contain the equivalent of a quarter cup of nuts. Since there's butter, yogurt, and eggs in the loaf, each slice has some additional calories. By slicing this dense and delicious loaf thin (20 slices), you get all the flavor of the bread with a very reasonable number of calories. This makes a great snack, breakfast toast, or accompaniment to a soup or stew.

You can get this bread into the oven in ten minutes, and it doesn't require a mixer. That's a good deal, since there's not much mess to clean up afterward.

Makes one 3½" x 7" loaf

3 eggs
1 cup plain, unsweetened yogurt
¼ cup melted butter
1 tsp. baking soda
½ tsp. salt
1 tsp. turmeric
3 cups almond flour
½ cup golden flaxseed meal

Preheat the oven to 350 degrees. Spray a loaf pan with some avocado or coconut oil.

In a mixing bowl, whisk the eggs; and then stir in the yogurt, melted butter, baking soda, salt, and turmeric. Fold in the almond flour and flaxseed meal. Pour the batter into the oiled loaf pan, and bake for about 45 minutes, until the loaf is fragrant, crusty, and brown. Store in the refrigerator for up to a week.

DR. J'S OMEGA-3 FOCACCIA BREAD

You've heard of Johnny Bread—now there's Joanie Bread! Gordon and I use this focaccia bread to go with meals on occasion or as a basis for pizza or open-faced sandwiches. If you spoon a little marinara sauce on it and cover it with a slice of mozzarella, you've got a tasty lunch.

Serves 10–12

4 eggs
¼ cup olive oil
1 4-oz. tub unsweetened, organic applesauce
1 tsp. baking powder
¾ tsp. salt
1 tsp. turmeric
1 cup almond flour
1 cup flaxseed meal
1 Tbsp. caraway seeds
Celtic sea salt (optional)

Preheat the oven to 350 degrees.

Whisk together the eggs and olive oil until they're well blended, and then beat in the applesauce. In a separate bowl, combine the dry ingredients (except for the caraway seeds and sea salt), and then add the wet ingredients to them. Let the dough sit in the bowl for five minutes to firm up.

Spray a cookie sheet or pizza pan with olive oil, and spread out the dough with your fingers into a thin rectangle or circle. Sprinkle with caraway seeds and sea salt, or any other spices you'd prefer.

Bake for 35 to 40 minutes until brown and crisp. Use a metal spatula to lift up the focaccia carefully around the edges and free the middle. I prefer to cut it in half—it's easier to free the two halves from the baking sheet. Cool the bread on a wire rack, and store it in a BPA-free plastic bag in the refrigerator. It will last for a week or more.

GRISELDA'S SEED CRACKERS

Sometimes when I'm just sitting around, minding my own business, or waking up in the morning, my food muse (I call her *Griselda*) drops in for an unexpected visit. Visions of yummy things then begin to dance in my mind. I've learned to write down what Griselda shares with me. These tasty seed crackers, with a crisp crunch, were one of her suggestions. If you like these as much as Gordon and I do, you can double the recipe.

Makes about 20 crackers

1 egg
2 Tbsp. melted butter
½ tsp. salt
¼ tsp. turmeric
½ tsp. baking powder
½ cup almond flour
¼ cup flaxseed meal
2 Tbsp. chia seeds
2 Tbsp. raw or toasted sunflower seeds

Preheat the oven to 375 degrees. Beat the egg with a wire whisk and then beat in the melted butter, salt, turmeric, and baking powder. Add the dry ingredients, stirring well. The mixture will be wet, so let it sit for five minutes. Then with clean hands, roll one-inch balls of dough, and press them thin and flat onto a greased cookie sheet. The dough won't spread out too much, so you can put them close together.

Bake for 10 to 12 minutes, and let cool on a wire rack. The crackers store well in a glass container (you can get the wide-mouthed cookie-jar type in Target) for up to a week.

TOASTED-SESAME CRACKERS

I adapted this tasty cracker recipe from Elana Amsterdam's *Paleo Cooking from Elana's Pantry,* a gluten-free, grain-free, and dairy-free cookbook. Elana is a wonderful baker and cook! The crackers were a bit bland for my taste, though, so I toasted the sesame seeds and added toasted sesame oil for a big flavor punch.

Makes about three-dozen crackers

½ cup sesame seeds
1 egg
1 Tbsp. toasted sesame oil
½ tsp. salt
1 cup almond flour

Preheat the oven to 350 degrees. Heat a skillet over medium heat, and add the sesame seeds, stirring them continuously for a couple of minutes until they turn light brown and fragrant. Scoop them out of the pan right away so they don't burn, and then spread them on a plate to cool completely before using in this recipe. (Tip: You can make a cup of the toasted seeds, then put the rest in a glass jar and use them to sprinkle on salads and vegetables. Delish.)

Whisk together the egg, sesame oil, and salt. Stir in the toasted sesame seeds and almond flour. Let the dough rest for five minutes, and then split it into portions. Roll each one into a ball between your hands, and then place it between two pieces of parchment paper. Roll it thin—the dough is amazingly sturdy. Take off the top piece of parchment, slide onto a cookie sheet, and cut the rolled dough into 1½-inch squares. You can bake them right on the parchment paper, but make sure that you use bleach-free paper. Bake for 10 to 12 minutes until toasty brown, but not burned.

PANCAKES WITH BLUEBERRY SAUCE

Gordon and I love blueberry muffins. Fortunately, *Wheat Belly*, by William Davis, has a great recipe for tender, delectable muffins that come out of the oven fragrant and perfectly browned.

One Sunday morning, we used those blueberry muffins as inspiration and created our version in the form of pancakes. You can whip these up and enjoy them in just a few minutes. Top them with blueberry sauce in place of syrup.

Serves 4

1 Tbsp. melted butter or coconut oil
2 eggs
⅔ cup yogurt, milk, or nut milk
1 cup blanched almond flour
¼ tsp. baking soda

Whisk together the wet ingredients, add the dry, and see what you've got. You may need to add a little more liquid depending on whether you prefer thick or thin pancakes. When you've reached the desired consistency, fry them up on a cast-iron griddle that you've greased with a little coconut oil. When the bubbles on the pancakes start to pop and the underside is brown, flip them over, and cook for another minute or two.

BLUEBERRY SAUCE

We used to love pancakes with real maple syrup, but what do you do if you don't want to eat all that concentrated sugar? Simple! Make a sugar-free fruit sauce. It's great served hot. Leftover sauce is delicious by itself or as a topping for sliced apples or other fruit.

Makes 2 cups

2 cups fresh or frozen blueberries
Truvia or other sweetener, to taste
2 tsp. lemon juice
½ tsp. cardamom or cinnamon, if desired

Mix all the ingredients in a glass bowl, microwave it for two minutes, and stir. If the berries have formed a sauce, you're good to go. If not, cook them a little bit longer.

KEEP-'EM-COMING CHOCOLATE-CHIP COOKIES

My husband waxes eloquent about how delicious these cookies are: "The best ever! Anywhere! Keep 'em coming." Yes, he's seriously prejudiced. And since he doesn't bake—and there aren't any store-bought cookies suitable for our lifestyle—my cookies are the only game in town, which gives me a definite competitive advantage. But I'd have to agree with Gordon—these are amazingly tasty cookies. The melt-in-your-mouth crunch, the mouthfeel, the nutty taste . . . oh, yes, you'll love 'em!

Makes 16–20 three-inch cookies

2 eggs
¼ cup melted coconut oil
2 tsp. vanilla
2 Tbsp. Truvia (or other stevia of preference)
½ tsp. baking soda
1 tsp. cinnamon
1 tsp. ground ginger
1½ cups almond flour
⅓ cup coarsely chopped raw walnuts
⅓ cup (heaping) organic dark-chocolate chips

Preheat the oven to 350 degrees. Using a wire whisk, beat the eggs until frothy. Add the melted coconut oil and keep whisking. Next add the vanilla, Truvia, baking soda, cinnamon, and ginger, again whisking to incorporate. Mix in the almond flour; then fold in the walnuts and chocolate chips. Let it sit for five minutes.

Spray a cookie pan with coconut or avocado oil. Spoon out heaping teaspoonfuls of dough, and roll them into balls—a task most kids would be more than eager to help with. Press each ball flat onto the baking sheet. (If you spray your hands first with some coconut oil, the process is much easier.) Bake for about 15 minutes, until the cookies are brown and fragrant, and move to a wire rack.

Tip: Wait until the cookies have cooled before you eat them. Their taste and texture changes as they cool down and crisp up.

Note on chocolate chips: A third of a cup of these tasty morsels contains only about 12 net grams of carbs; 1½ cups of ground almonds (the flour) contain 12 net carbs; and the one-third cup of chopped nuts adds another 2 or 3 net carbs. This works out to just a gram or two of carbs per cookie—but pay attention! These cookies are way low in carbs, but they still have calories. After all, they're made of nuts and oil. So although it's tempting to eat several in a sitting, two make a healthy snack that will help fill you up and keep you satisfied because of the protein content in the nuts and the satiety factor of the fat.

THUMBPRINT COOKIES

The first time I made these cookies, Gordon outdid himself in the compliment department. He declared these the best cookies ever, beating out even his former favorite—my chocolate-chip cookies. I make these often and agree that they're incredibly fragrant, tender, and satiating.

Makes 20 small cookies

1 egg
2 Tbsp. coconut oil or melted butter
1 tsp. vanilla
¼ tsp. salt

½ tsp. baking soda
1 tsp. cinnamon
1 tsp. ginger
1 Tbsp. Truvia
1 cup almond flour
¼ cup chopped walnuts
2–3 Tbsp. pure fruit jam

Preheat the oven to 350 degrees. In a mixing bowl, beat the egg until frothy, and add the melted coconut oil or butter. Whisk in the vanilla, salt, baking soda, spices, and Truvia; then fold in the almond flour and walnuts.

With clean hands, roll small balls of dough and place them on a cookie sheet sprayed with coconut or avocado oil. Make a thumbprint indentation in each cookie. For the sake of efficiency, roll all the dough into balls first, then go down the sheet, making the thumbprints. Fill each cookie with about a half teaspoon of jam, and bake for about 15 minutes. Let cool on a wire rack. Not many carbs there, but lots of flavor!

COCONUT-AMBROSIA COOKIES

If you like coconut, you'll appreciate the chewy morsels that make these cookies so satisfying to eat. They are incredibly light, tender, and filled with coconut goodness. They're good for your brain as well. And—what else would you expect?—these are also Gordon's favorite cookies. He's a two-timing, no, a three-timing cookie man. Hands down, these are my absolute favorite cookies, too!

Makes 30 cookies

2 eggs
1 tsp. vanilla
Dash of salt
1 tsp. baking soda
½ cup melted coconut oil

1 cup almond flour
1 cup unsweetened, organic coconut flakes
¼ cup (heaping) dark-chocolate chips

Preheat the oven to 350 degrees. Grease a cookie sheet with a coconut-oil spray, or rub some coconut oil onto the sheet with a paper towel.

Beat the eggs with a wire whisk, and then beat in the vanilla, salt, baking soda, and melted coconut oil. Add the almond flour, and then fold in the coconut flakes and chocolate chips.

Let the dough sit for five minutes to thicken up, and then drop onto the greased cookie sheet, flattening the cookies slightly. Bake for about 15 minutes until lightly browned, and let cool on a wire rack.

Desserts and Snacks

BERRY-CHERRY GEL-YO

Growing up, no family feast was complete without a fluorescent red, orange, green, or yellow sugary Jello mold studded with canned fruit. It's amazing that we didn't all glow in the dark. My Gel-Yo is a whole different beast. It's orgasmically delicious, beautiful to behold, and downright good for you. While gelatin (pure collagen) isn't a complete protein, it contains about half the essential amino acids needed for life. It's digested into short peptides called *glyprolines* that are healing for the gut. The authors of a 2010 article concluded that "glyprolines hold much promise as pharmaceutical products, which can be used in gastroenterological practice for the prevention and therapy of ulcer disease of the stomach and duodenum."[3]

Serves 8

2 cups frozen bing cherries
1 cup frozen blueberries
Water
2 Tbsp. unflavored gelatin (I use Grass Valley, kosher and halal from grass-fed cows.)
½ tsp. cardamom
2 Tbsp. Truvia

Put the fruit into a four-cup glass measuring cup, and add enough water to fill to the 3½-cup line. Add contents to a saucepan and bring to a boil, allowing it to simmer for a few minutes to release the fruit juices. In a small bowl, dissolve the gelatin in a half cup of cold water and add it to the hot stuff. Add the cardamom and Truvia. Stir and pour into a bowl or individual ramekins. Chill until set—about four hours.

Variations: Add a half cup yogurt (cow's milk, goat's milk, or soy milk) in place of the same volume of water. You can also experiment with different combinations of berries or other fruits. Boil the fruit first according to the recipe, both to free the natural fruit juices that make the gelatin so delicious, and, in the case of cherries and berries, to make them deeply colorful. Many kinds of fresh fruit contain enzymes that prevent the chemical reaction that causes a gel to set. These are inactivated by boiling.

HEAVENLY BAKED APPLES

I used to core apples and bake them whole, but that changed when Gordon and I rented a house in Taos, New Mexico, for two weeks. I packed up a box of kitchen utensils, but forgot the apple corer, so I just quartered the apples instead. It was so easy and tasty that I never went back to baking whole apples. It's also nice to have the flexibility of eating just a quarter or a half an apple—they make a great garnish.

Serves 4–8

4 Granny Smith apples quartered, with the cores removed
½–1 cup cherries or blueberries
1 cup water
1 tsp. ground cinnamon
½ tsp. ground cardamom
½ tsp. ground ginger
1 Tbsp. Truvia

Preheat the oven to 375 degrees. Put the quartered apples in an ovenproof glass dish, and pour the cherries or blueberries around them. In a saucepan bring the water to a boil, and stir in the spices and Truvia. Then pour the mixture over the fruit. Cover and bake for about an hour. There will still be water in the bottom of this dish when you take it out of the oven, but after the apples sit for about an hour, most of the water will be absorbed, leaving just a nice bit of syrup.

FRUIT AND NUTS DIPPED IN CHOCOLATE

This is my favorite dessert. It's so easy that you can have it on the table in just a few minutes.

Serves any number

Strawberries
Apples, cut in chunks
Other fruits of your choice
Nuts of your choice
Dark chocolate sauce

Put 2 tablespoons of chocolate sauce per serving into the microwave, if you use one, or warm it on the stove. There are a lot of delicious brands out there of organic, fair-trade sauce. Make sure to choose dark chocolate, and read the label to avoid sauces that are high in carbs. The good ones have just a few carbs per serving. Put the bowl of warm chocolate, sliced fruit, and nuts on a festive plate—and go to town.

POPCORN

While we generally don't eat grains, organic nonGMO popcorn is an occasional exception. I adapted this recipe from one found on the Internet a few years ago. It's great because virtually every kernel pops. If you're having company or a party for a child, a popcorn bar is festive and fun. You can easily triple the recipe as long as you use a big pot so that every kernel has space, and they don't bunch up.

Serves 3–4

⅓ cup organic nonGMO popcorn
3 Tbsp. coconut oil
Sea salt or other spices to taste

Heat the oil for a few minutes in a six-quart pot over medium-high heat. Add two to three kernels of popcorn, cover the pot, and wait for them to pop. This lets you know when the oil is at the right heat. Turn the heat down to medium, add the popcorn, and cover. Shake occasionally, and it will soon start to pop, which will happen pretty much all at once. Pour it into a big bowl, salt and season to taste, and mix it up well.

For fun, serve portions of popcorn in individual bowls and set up a toppings bar. Choose from condiments such as:

Grated Parmesan cheese
Black pepper
Cinnamon
Cocoa powder
Nutritional yeast
Turmeric
Curry powder
Chili powder
Herbes de Provence
Rosemary

CRUNCHY KALE CHIPS

The first few times I tried to make kale chips, they came out burned and bitter. When Marilyn Tam shared her recipe with me, the results were way better. The secret was to use a much lower oven temperature.

Makes about 6 servings

1 bunch curly kale
2 Tbsp. olive oil
Sea salt and pepper to taste
Sesame seeds (optional)
Sesame oil (optional)

Preheat the oven to 300 degrees. Wash kale; dry thoroughly in a salad spinner; and tear into bite-size pieces, removing the center stems and saving them for other uses. Toss kale pieces with olive oil, rubbing the leaves with your hands to make sure each gets a coating of oil so they crisp up well. You can add more oil if needed, but in this case, less is more. Add sea salt, pepper, sesame seeds, and a few drops of sesame oil, if desired, to taste.

Place kale in a single layer on an oiled baking sheet(s). Bake for 12 to 15 minutes, checking frequently to make sure it doesn't burn. Remove pieces as they crisp up, to allow the remaining kale chips to get even heat.

Dressings, Sauces, and Marinades

DR. J'S KICKIN' SPICE MIX

This mix of antioxidant, anti-inflammatory spices is delicious. By making it up in batches, you simplify food preparation since you only have to measure out one ingredient instead of eight in subsequent uses. There's not enough chili to make this really hot—just enough to perk up the flavors and make hearty dishes more satisfying (unless you decide to kick it up a notch by adding more chili powder). It's great in soups, stews, and stir-fries.

2 Tbsp. powdered turmeric
2 Tbsp. ground cumin
2 Tbsp. ground coriander
2 Tbsp. ground ginger
2 Tbsp. ground chili (more if you like it hot)
1 Tbsp. ground cardamom
1 Tbsp. ground cinnamon
1 Tbsp. garlic salt

Mix the spices together, and store in a glass jar. Try adding a small amount of this (start with a half teaspoon) to your cooking oil when you're stir-frying vegetables. If you like it, add more to taste. It's spicy, so you won't want to use it all the time, but in moderation, it creates fragrant, savory dishes that make you a standout chef. I suggest adding the spice mix to your cooking oil (typical in Indian cooking) because the phytochemicals in many of these spices aren't water soluble; rather, they need to combine with oil to become more bioavailable.

SUPER BOWL HOT-WING SAUCE

Gordon was going to a Super Bowl party. I was finishing this book and stayed home to write, but I did send him off with three dozen hot wings after saving a few for myself. It took about a half cup of the sauce in this recipe to coat the wings before baking at 400 degrees, turning frequently, for about half an hour. I used some of the leftover sauce to coat fillets of frozen (then thawed and squeezed) tofu. The freezing gives it a chewier texture. Pretty good, actually.

Makes 1¼ cups

¼ cup extra-virgin olive oil
¼ cup vegan Worcestershire sauce
2 Tbsp. apple-cider vinegar (I use Bragg's.)
2 Tbsp. gluten-free soy sauce
½ cup organic, sugar-free ketchup
1 tsp. turmeric
1 Tbsp. ground chili pepper
1 tsp. ground star anise
½ tsp. Truvia
½ tsp. (heaping) salt
Hot sauce of your choice to taste (optional, to kick up the heat)

Combine all the ingredients in a recycled glass jar, and shake it up well. It will last in the refrigerator for a month or longer.

MARINADE FOR GRILLING

Marinating meat inhibits the formation of cancer-causing chemicals that form when meat is cooked over high heat or grilled. Also, marinating your protein—whether it's vegetable or animal protein—makes it tastier and opens up a whole world of flavor. Here's a simple recipe that works well. Gordon adapted it from *Bon Appétit*'s cookbook *Fast, Easy, Fresh*.

Juice of one lemon
One clove garlic
1 tsp. herbes de Provence
2 tsp. capers
¼ cup olive oil

Put the ingredients in a blender or food processor, and whiz them up. Marinate foods for at least 20 minutes prior to grilling.

GORDON'S VINAIGRETTE DRESSING

Gordon is the dressing maker in our household. His vinaigrette is so good that we rarely use anything else. I can't even begin to imagine why anyone would buy dressing in bottles when it's so much tastier and more economical to make your own. It takes just a few minutes.

Makes 10 ounces

¾ cup extra-virgin olive oil (the best you can afford)
½ cup white balsamic vinegar
1 tsp. good-quality mustard
½ tsp. Truvia
Salt and pepper to taste

Put all the ingredients in a recycled glass jar and shake until blended. You can vary this endlessly by adding minced garlic, fresh or dried herbs, paprika, or whatever rings your bell. The secret is the fine fragrant oil, the white balsamic, and the ratio between them (3:2). Remember that ratio for a perfect vinaigrette every time.

That's All, Folks!

I hope you enjoy experimenting with this ragtag collection of recipes. For more ideas, the Internet affords a wealth of possibilities, of course. A few good cookbooks to have on hand, though, either for the actual recipes or for the inspiration, are as follows:

- *True Food*, by Andrew Weil, M.D., Sam Fox, and Michael Stebner. Andy really knows and loves food. He's a brilliant ethnobotanist, a great doc, and a masterful chef. This is a book of gourmet recipes from his True Food restaurant chain.

- *Fast, Easy, Fresh*, by *Bon Appétit*. The title sums it up. It's our go-to book.

- *Wheat Belly*, by William Davis, M.D. The source of the world's best almond-flour blueberry muffins.

- *The South Beach Diet Supercharged*, by Arthur Agatston, M.D. Simple meal plans and good recipes that are easily adapted to a PlantPlus Diet.

- *My Kitchen Cure*, by Mee Tracy McCormick. Just reading about Mee's journey of recovery from autoimmune disease is a recipe for inspiration. The food recipes are good, too, especially if your diet sleuthing leads you to eat grains and beans.

Now that you know what to eat, continuing to personalize your diet and finding the foods that you really love will keep you mindful, healthy, and creative. But until you're ready to do the Reboot and Personalization, you might just want to use these recipes to go PlantPlus *Lite*. Instructions for that are in the next chapter.

CHAPTER 28

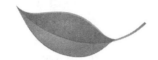

PlantPlus Lite:

A Few Changes Go a Long Way

*"You don't have to see the whole staircase.
Just take the first step."*

— MARTIN LUTHER KING, JR.

Since you've read through some of or even all this nutritional tome, you're obviously interested in changing the way you eat. Thank you so much for allowing me to be part of your journey. Whatever you take from this book, and whatever you leave, let your own wise self be your guide. If you're ready to take the leap, then trying the whole PlantPlus program may be right for you. If not, you can still make a major difference to your health and well-being with just a few adjustments to your diet. That's what this last chapter is about.

Let me tell you the story of a woman who made a big shift with a few simple changes.

I had plans to meet up with my friend Laura, and it had been a couple of years since we'd last seen each other in person. Laura is a tall woman—I'd say 5'8"—and was always a little on the hefty side, maybe a size 14 or 16. I looked around the restaurant where we'd agreed to meet and couldn't locate her, although the hostess said that she'd already arrived. Finally, after a few minutes of searching, I spied an eager hand waving across the room. A tall, very slender woman (perhaps a size 8) with long hair (Laura's had always been short) was standing up, smiling, and beckoning me to join her.

It's not often that a change in someone's appearance leaves you flabbergasted. But Laura's transformation was so off the charts that I had to keep forcing myself to look away for fear of staring rudely. That was over five years ago, and she hasn't gained back a pound.

Naturally, I asked Laura how she did it.

"I made just one change," she confided. "I eliminated everything that has flour in it."

Laura was known for her fabulous baking, particularly her pies. "What do you do now that you can't make piecrusts?" I asked. Her new specialty turned out to be crisps—using a little oatmeal and a lot of nuts to top different types of fruit.

One little dietary change literally reshaped Laura's life.

Pareto's Principle: Why Small Changes Go a Long Way

Pareto's Principle is also known as the 80/20 rule. Italian economist Vilfredo Pareto observed back in 1906 that 80 percent of the peas in his vegetable garden grew in 20 percent of the pods. His observation was gradually extended to suggest that 80 percent of results (whether you're a car salesman, a marketing guru, or perhaps someone following a diet) come from 20 percent of the effort you make. For example, if you aren't up for committing to a total PlantPlus makeover, you can still come a long way just by making a few changes. I call this program PlantPlus Lite.

PlantPlus Lite

1. Eliminate anything containing "white foods," such as sugar and flour, including gluten-free products.

2. Eat a pound of vegetables every day and a couple of whole fruits for good measure.

If you make these two simple changes, you're quite likely to improve your health and lose weight.

I wish you well on your journey.

Epilogue

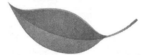

The Cheshire Cat

*"Oh what a grin, it's nearly a sin
to have your cake and eat it, too.
But you finally can
with your own PlantPlus plan.
So eat well,
and enjoy the win-win."*

— FROM JOAN IN WONDERLAND

Yes, I know that rhyme is corny beyond belief, but what's life without being mad as a hatter now and again?

PlantPlus is a way of life that entertains, inspires, and brings out the best in us. Eating consciously changes everything, because food is ubiquitous. When we do food differently—getting out of old behavioral ruts—our mental energy flows into new brain circuits. We slowly begin to rewire our habits with regard to the most intimate and dominant experience of our lives: eating.

You win because you get healthier in body and mind. You help the environment, farmworkers who deserve a fair wage, and of course, your children and your children's children. This is all better than nice, but if that were all that a PlantPlus Diet did, most people wouldn't be able to stick with it. The bottom line is that it's delicious and fun.

Writing this book has helped Gordon and me with the evolution of our own diet. Your nutritional journey, of course, is likely to be quite different than our own. As we discussed in the Introduction, we're each metabolically unique, and one man's or woman's food is another person's poison.

We began our campaign to improve our health with a high-carb, low-fat, near-vegan diet that wreaked havoc with Gordon's blood lipids and my blood pressure. Both of us also gained weight. Next we initiated a low-carb, near-Paleo program—lots of vegetables, nuts, and meats—but we also included dairy. The result was stupendous in almost every way. We lost weight, lost our aches and pains, and Gordon's triglyceride levels fell while his good HDL cholesterol levels rose.

Then, after about a year, we discovered that despite the many benefits of our low-carb, high-fat regime, both of us had an unexpected result. Our LDL-P, total cholesterol particle number—a strong predictor of heart disease—was elevated. As a result, we cut back substantially on meat and hard cheese. We're not vegans now by a long shot, but our sleuthing has led to a diet that's almost all plants, with the Plus additions of a little soft cheese, fish, poultry, and nonfat yogurt. Now meat's a cheat rather than a mainstay.

Your diet is likely to evolve over time as well if you keep track of your food, mood, well-being, and lab tests. As a result you'll become more mindful about how foods affect you. That mindfulness will spread to the rest of your life, too, reducing stress and increasing happiness.

Because we're partners in this health journey, Gordon and I have been brought even closer by our nutritional experiments. We frequently shop and cook together, inventing new dishes and enjoying old favorites. Rather than being a chore, cooking has become a source of joy.

It's early spring as I complete this book, and the Boulder farmers' market will soon open again. I can almost taste those fresh greens. We love to wander through the stalls, picking out produce and saying hello to friends who are also shopping there.

I hope that you'll find a partner—whether it's a friend, a lover, or a spouse—to share this way of life with you. PlantPlus is as much a relationship evolution as what cardiologist Steven R. Gundry calls a *diet evolution.*

The foods that make up the core of PlantPlus are deeply nourishing. They make you feel contented, a bit excited, and always ready to be surprised. So have the time of your life. PlantPlus is a juicy, creative lifestyle for people who want to enjoy themselves while maximizing their health and well-being. I hope that's You.

Thanks for reading this book.

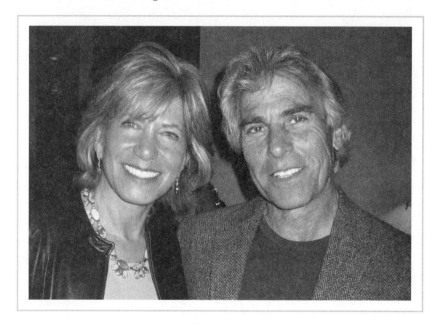

You can join the lively conversation on my Facebook page: www.facebook.com/joanborysenkocommunity. And please stop by my website, www.joanborysenko.com, for more tips on living a PlantPlus life.

Appendix

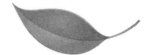

MEDICAL SYMPTOM CHECKLIST (MSCL)

Hi again, dear reader. It's a good idea for you to make several copies of this form so that you'll always have one ready before and after a diet change. Then you'll have a baseline for comparison.

Indicate how often you've had any of the following medical symptoms during *the past month.*

	Never/ Almost Never	Rarely	Some-times	Often	Always/ Almost Always
1. Blurred or double vision not corrected by glasses	0	1	2	3	4
2. Numbness or tingling	0	1	2	3	4
3. Sudden feelings of weakness or faintness	0	1	2	3	4
4. Any infections, irritations, or pains in the eyes or ears	0	1	2	3	4
5. Nasal or sinus discharge or stuffiness (stuffy or runny nose)	0	1	2	3	4

	Never/ Almost Never	Rarely	Some- times	Often	Always/ Almost Always
6. Shortness of breath even after light work	0	1	2	3	4
7. Cough at any time, day or night	0	1	2	3	4
8. Sore throat or runny nose with a fever as high as 100° for at least two days	0	1	2	3	4
9. Frequent headaches	0	1	2	3	4
10. Palpitations (heart pounding or racing, irregular heartbeats)	0	1	2	3	4
11. Repeated pain in or near the heart (chest pain)	0	1	2	3	4
12. Cold hands or feet	0	1	2	3	4
13. Frequent backaches	0	1	2	3	4
14. Muscle aches or pain in shoulders, neck, or limbs	0	1	2	3	4
15. Waking up with stiff, swollen, or aching joints	0	1	2	3	4
16. Rash or itching skin	0	1	2	3	4
17. Sensitive or tender skin	0	1	2	3	4
18. Excessive sweating	0	1	2	3	4
19. Diarrhea or constipation	0	1	2	3	4
20. Repeated indigestion, heartburn, or upset stomach	0	1	2	3	4
21. Vomiting	0	1	2	3	4

	Never/ Almost Never	Rarely	Some- times	Often	Always/ Almost Always
22. Nausea	0	1	2	3	4
23. Abdominal pains (pains or cramps in the belly or gut)	0	1	2	3	4
24. Difficulty swallowing	0	1	2	3	4
25. Frequent urination, or pain or pressure with urination	0	1	2	3	4
26. Vaginal symptoms (discharge, itching, burning, odor, infection)	0	1	2	3	4
27. Vaginal bleeding	0	1	2	3	4
28. Low sexual desire	0	1	2	3	4
29. Painful intercourse	0	1	2	3	4
30. Pelvic pain	0	1	2	3	4
31. Rectal bleeding	0	1	2	3	4
32. Difficulty sleeping (insomnia)	0	1	2	3	4
33. Feeling tired or fatigued even with usual amounts of rest	0	1	2	3	4
34. Loss of appetite	0	1	2	3	4
35. Other symptom (specify: _____)	0	1	2	3	4

Conversion Charts

Standard Cup	Fine Powder (e.g., flour)	Grain (e.g., rice)	Granular (e.g., sugar)	Liquid Solids (e.g., butter)	Liquid (e.g., milk)
1	140 g	150 g	190 g	200 g	240 ml
¾	105 g	113 g	143 g	150 g	180 ml
⅔	93 g	100 g	125 g	133 g	160 ml
½	70 g	75 g	95 g	100 g	120 ml
⅓	47 g	50 g	63 g	67 g	80 ml
¼	35 g	38 g	48 g	50 g	60 ml
⅛	18 g	19 g	24 g	25 g	30 ml

Useful Equivalents for Liquid Ingredients by Volume				
¼ tsp				1 ml
½ tsp				2 ml
1 tsp				5 ml
3 tsp	1 tbsp		½ fl oz	15 ml
	2 tbsp	⅛ cup	1 fl oz	30 ml
	4 tbsp	¼ cup	2 fl oz	60 ml
	5⅓ tbsp	⅓ cup	3 fl oz	80 ml
	8 tbsp	½ cup	4 fl oz	120 ml
	10⅔ tbsp	⅔ cup	5 fl oz	160 ml
	12 tbsp	¾ cup	6 fl oz	180 ml
	16 tbsp	1 cup	8 fl oz	240 ml
	1 pt	2 cups	16 fl oz	480 ml
	1 qt	4 cups	32 fl oz	960 ml
			33 fl oz	1000 ml	1 liter

Useful Equivalents for Dry Ingredients by Weight

(To convert ounces to grams, multiply the number of ounces by 30.)

1 oz	¹⁄₁₆ lb	30 g
4 oz	¼ lb	120 g
8 oz	½ lb	240 g
12 oz	¾ lb	360 g
16 oz	1 lb	480 g

Useful Equivalents for Cooking/Oven Temperatures

Process	Fahrenheit	Celsius	Gas Mark
Freeze Water	32° F	0° C	
Room Temperature	68° F	20° C	
Boil Water	212° F	100° C	
Bake	325° F	160° C	3
	350° F	180° C	4
	375° F	190° C	5
	400° F	200° C	6
	425° F	220° C	7
	450° F	230° C	8
Broil			Grill

Useful Equivalents for Length

(To convert inches to centimeters, multiply the number of inches by 2.5.)

1 in			2.5 cm	
6 in	½ ft		15 cm	
12 in	1 ft		30 cm	
36 in	3 ft	1 yd	90 cm	
40 in			100 cm	1 m

Endnotes

Introduction

1. Rosenberg, D.; "Diet Advice from Israel: Eat Your Vegetables," 3/07/12. www.jpost.com/Health-and-Science/Diet-advice-from-Israel-Eat -your-vegetables.

2. Canfi, A. et al.; "Effect of Changes in the Intake of Weight of Specific Food Groups on Successful Body Weight Loss During a Multi–Dietary Strategy Intervention Trial," *Journal of the American College of Nutrition,* 2011; 30(6): 491–501.

3. Liebman, B.; "New Clues to Weight Gain and Loss: Is One Diet More Effective Than Another for Weight Loss?" 2/12/2014. www .nutritionaction.com/daily/diet-and-weight-loss/new-clues-to -weight-gain-and-loss.

Chapter 1

1. Taubes, G.; *Why We Get Fat and What to Do About It.* New York: Anchor Books, Random House, 2011.

2. "Economic Costs of Diabetes in the U.S. in 2012," American Diabetes Association, Diabetes Care, April 2013; 36(4):1,033–1,046. http://care.diabetesjournals.org/content/36/4/1033.full.

Chapter 2

1. Smith-Spangler, C. et al.; "Are Organic Foods Safer or Healthier Than Conventional Alternatives? A Systematic Review," *Annals of Internal Medicine,* Sept 2012; 157(5):348–366.

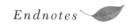

2. "What Is Inflammation? What Causes Inflammation?" www.medicalnewstoday.com/articles/248423.php.

3. Gundry, S.R.; *Dr. Gundry's Diet Evolution*. New York: Three Rivers Press, Random House, 2008.

4. Vasdev, S. et al; "Role of Advanced Glycation End Products in Hypertension and Atherosclerosis: Therapeutic Implications," *Cell Biochem Biophys*, 2007; 49(1):48–63.

5. Pollan, M.; "Some of My Best Friends Are Germs," www.nytimes .com/2013/05/19/magazine/say-hello-to-the-100-trillion-bacteria -that-make-up-your-microbiome.html?pagewanted=all&_r=0.

6. Thomas, L; *The Lives of a Cell: Notes of a Biology Watcher*, 1974.

7. Sommer, F. et al; "The Gut Microbiota—Masters of Host Development and Physiology," *Nature Reviews Microbiology* 11, April 2013:227–238. doi:10.1038/nrmicro2974.

Chapter 4

1. Hamblin, J.; "This Is Your Brain on Gluten," *The Atlantic*, Dec. 20, 2013. www.theatlantic.com/health/archive/2013/12/this-is-your -brain-on-gluten/282550/.

2. Feinman, R.D.; "Saturated Fat and Health: Recent Advances in Research Lipids," October 2010; 45(10):891–892. Published online September 9, 2010. doi: 10.1007/s11745-010-3446-8.

3. Kresser, C.; "The Diet-Heart Myth," http://my.chriskresser.com /wp-content/uploads/membership-files/ebooks/Diet%20Heart%20 Myth.pdf.

4. Siri-Tarino, P.W. et al; "Meta-Analysis of Prospective Cohort Studies Evaluating the Association of Saturated Fat with Cardiovascular Disease," *Am J Clin Nutr*, Mar 2010; 91(3):535–46. doi: 10.3945/ajcn .2009.27725. Epub 2010 Jan 13.

5. Attia, P.; The Eating Academy, glossary for *triglycerides*.

Chapter 5

1. Porter, N.; "FDA Aims to Eliminate Artificial Trans Fats," www .washingtontimes.com/news/2013/nov/7/fda-aims-eliminate -artificial-trans-fats/?page=all.

2. Field, C.J. et al.; "Human Health Benefits of Vaccenic Acid," *Appl Physiol Nutr Metab*, Oct 2009; 34(5):979–91. doi: 10.1139/H09-079.

3. "Profiling Food Consumption in America," www.usda.gov /factbook/chapter2.pdf.

4. Dalleau, S. et al; "Cell death and diseases related to oxidative stress:4-hydroxynonenal (HNE) in the balance," *Cell Death & Differentiation 20*, Dec 2013:1,615–1,630. doi:10.1038/cdd.2013.13ARTICLE T.

5. "Cotton and the Environment," www.ota.com/organic/environment /cotton_environment.html.

Chapter 6

1. Ramsden, C.E. et al; "Use of dietary linoleic acid for secondary prevention of coronary heart disease and death: evaluation of recovered data from the Sydney Diet Heart Study and updated meta-analysis," *BMJ*, Feb 2013; 346:e8707. doi: 10.1136/bmj.e8707.

2. *Science Daily,* "Study Raises Questions About Dietary Fats and Heart Disease," Feb. 5, 2013. www.sciencedaily.com /releases/2013/02/130205200239.htm.

3. "What Are the Health Benefit of Olive Oil?" www.medicalnewstoday .com/articles/266258.php.

Chapter 7

1. Freed, D J.; "Do Dietary Lectins Cause Disease?" *BMJ*, 1999; 318. doi: http://dx.doi.org/10.1136/bmj.318.7190.1023 (Published April 17,1999).

2. Kresser, C.; "50 Shades of Gluten Intolerance," 4/03/2013. www .huffingtonpost.com/chris-kresser/gluten-intolerance_b_2964812 .htm.

3. Hopkins, K.; "Dog Evolution Included Getting the Starch In," *Scientific American,* January 31, 2013.

Chapter 8

1. Dekker, M.J. et al; "Fructose: A Highly Lipogenic Nutrient Implicated in Insulin Resistance, Hepatic Steatosis, and the Metabolic Syndrome," *American Journal of Physiology: Endocrinology and Metabolism,* November 1, 2010; 299.

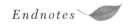

Chapter 9

1. Obici, S. et al; "Minireview: Nutrient Sensing and the Regulation of Insulin Action and Energy Balance," www.physiciansregional medicalgroup.com/health-education/85,P08342.

2. Jönsson, T. et al; "Agrarian Diet and Diseases of Affluence— Do Evolutionary Novel Dietary Lectins Cause Leptin Resistance?" www.biomedcentral.com/1472-6823/5/10.

Chapter 10

1. Freedman, D.H.; "Lies, Damned Lies. And Medical Science," *The Atlantic*, Oct 4, 2010. www.theatlantic.com/magazine /archive/2010/11/lies-damned-lies-and-medical-science/308269.

2. Koeth, R.A. et al; "Intestinal Microbiota Metabolism of L-Carnitine, a Nutrient in Red Meat, Promotes Atherosclerosis." *Nat Med*, May 2013; 19(5):576–85. doi: 10.1038/nm.3145. Epub 2013 Apr 7.

3. Leach, J.; "From Meat to Microbes to Main Street: Is It Time to Trade In Your George Foreman Grill?" The Human Food Project: Anthropology of Microbes, April 15, 2013. http://humanfoodproject.com /from-meat-to-microbes-to-main-street-is-it-time-to-trade-in-your -george-foreman-grill/From.

4. Bojigin, J. et al; "Surge of Neurophysiological Coherence and Connectivity in the Dying Brain," *Proc. Natl. Acad. Sci,* 2013; 110 (47) E4405.

5. Zheng, J.S. et al; "Intake of fish and marine n-3 polyunsaturated fatty acids and risk of breast cancer: meta-analysis of data from 21 independent prospective cohort studies,"*BMJ,* 2013:346:f3706.

6. Attia, P.; "What I Actually Eat: Part 3," (circa Q1 2013) http:// eatingacademy.com/personal/actually-eat-part-iii-circa-q1-2014.

Chapter 11

1. Gardner, C.D. et al; "Comparison of the Atkins, Zone, Ornish, and LEARN Diets for Change in Weight and Related Risk Factors Among Overweight Premenopausal Women: The A TO Z Weight Loss Study: A Randomized Trial." *JAMA,* 2007; 297(9):969–977. doi:10.1001/jama.297.9.969.

2. Gardner, C.; "The Battle of the Diets: Is Anyone Winning (at Losing?)," Stanford School of Medicine Medcast Lecture Series, May 22, 2008. www.youtube.com/watch?v=eREuZEdMAVo.

Chapter 12

1. Ebbeling, C.B. et al; "Effects of Dietary Composition on Energy Expenditure During Weight-Loss Maintenance," *JAMA*, 2012; 307(24):2627–2634. doi:10.1001/jama.2012.6607. Children's Hospital Boston (June 26, 2012).

2. "Dieting? Study Challenges Notion That a Calorie Is Just a Calorie," *ScienceDaily*. Retrieved July 18, 2013, from www.sciencedaily.com /releases/2012/06/120626163801.htm.

Chapter 13

1. "A to Z Study Follow Up: Collection of DNA Data from Buccal Swabs," http://clinicaltrials.gov/show/NCT00866151. Page 3 of 3.

2. Nelson, M.D. et al; "Genotype Patterns Predict Weight Loss Success: The Right Diet Does Matter," EPI|NPAM 2010; March 2–5, 2010, San Francisco, CA.

3. Information included in the Pathway Genomics Pathway Fit Diet, Nutrition, and Exercise personal genetic report (2012). 4045 Sorrento Valley Blvd., San Diego, CA 92121.

Chapter 14

1. "How Intestinal Bacteria May Make You Fat," *Newsweek* and The Daily Beast, www.thedailybeast.com/newsweek/2010/07/06/don-t -just-blame-calories.html. Page 1 of 4.

2. Ridaura, V.K. et al; "Gut Microbiota from Twins Discordant for Obesity Modulate Metabolism in Mice," *Science,* Sept 6, 2013; 341(6150):1241214. doi:10.1126/science.1241214.

3. Everard, A. et al; "Cross-Talk Between Akkermansia Muciniphila and Intestinal Epithelium Controls Diet-Induced Obesity," PNAS 2013; 110(22):9066-9071.

4. Maes, M. et al; "Increased IgA and IgM Responses Against Gut Commensals in Chronic Depression: Further Evidence for Increased Bacterial Translocation or Leaky Gut," *J Affect Disord,* Dec 1 2012; 141(1):55–62. doi: 10.1016/j.jad.2012.02.023. Epub Mar 11, 2012.

5. Leach, J.; "Can a High Fat Paleo Diet Cause Obesity and Diabetes? Maybe, Unless," Human Food Project, June 24, 2012. http:// humanfoodproject.com/can-a-high-fat-paleo-diet-cause-obesity-and -diabetes.

6. Ibid.

7. Van Nood, E. et al; "Duodenal Infusion of Donor Feces for Recurrent Clostridium Difficile," *N Engl J Med,* 2013; 368:407–41.

8. Vrieze, A.V. et al; "Transfer of Intestinal Microbiota from Lean Donors Increases Insulin Sensitivity in Individuals with Metabolic Syndrome," *Gastroenterology,* Oct 2012; 143(4):913–916.

9. Brown, A.; "The SAD Generation? Study Finds That Millennials Are Stressed Out and Depressed," Feb. 8, 2013, http://madamenoire .com/261687/the-sad-generation-study-finds-millennials-are -stressed-out-and-depressed/#sthash.glBvKx0z.dpuf.

10. Leach, J.; "Honor Thy Symbionts," Jeff D. Leach and Human Food Project, 2012:118.

11. Leach, J.; *Eat Bugs. Not Too Much. Mainly with Plants.* New Orleans, 2008: 16.

Chapter 15

1. Cronin, M.; "Junk Food Addiction Linked to Pregnant Mothers' Eating Habits, Research Says." www.huffingtonpost.com/2013/05/07/junk -food-addiction-pregnant-mothers_n_3186552.html.

2. Ong, Z.Y. et al; "Maternal 'Junk-Food' Feeding of Rat Dams Alters Food Choices and Development of the Mesolimbic Reward Pathway in the Offspring," FASEB J, Jul 2011; 25(7):2167–79. doi: 10.1096/fj.10-178392. Epub Mar 22, 2011.

3. Ibid.

4. Crews, D. et al; "Epigenetic Transgenerational Inheritance of Altered Stress Responses," PNAS 2012; published ahead of print May 21, 2012. doi:10.1073/pnas.1118514109.

5. Dolinoy, D.C., "The Agouti Mouse Model: An Epigenetic Biosensor for Nutritional and Environmental Alterations on the Fetal Epigenome," *Nutrition Reviews.* 66 (Supple. 1), 2008:S7-11.

Chapter 16

1. Attia, P.; The Eating Academy, http://eatingacademy.com/nutrition /gravity-and-insulin-the-dynamic-duo.

2. Attia, P.; The Eating Academy, http://eatingacademy.com/nutrition /if-low-carb-eating-is-so-effective-why-are-people-still-overweight.

3. Verekamp, N.; www.livestrong.com/article/227474-how-many-carbs -should-you-have-a-day-to-lose-weight/#ixzz2QTxYemzx. June 14 2011.

Chapter 17

1. Verekamp, N.; www.livestrong.com/article/227474-how-many-carbs -should-you-have-a-day-to-lose-weight/#ixzz2QTxYemzx. June 14, 2011.

2. "Get the facts: Sources of Sodium in Your Diet," www.cdc.gov/salt /pdfs/sources_of_sodium.pdf.

3. http://thechart.blogs.cnn.com/2010/08/05/about-60-percent-pay -attention-to-nutrition-facts.

Chapter 18

1. "The Hemoglobin A1c (HbA1c) test for Diabetes," WebMD, http://diabetes.webmd.com/guide/glycated-hemoglobin-test-hba1c.

Chapter 19

1. http://health.usnews.com/health-news/articles/2013/01/07/us-news -best-diets-how-we-rated-29-eating-plans.

Chapter 21

1. Jakubowicz, D.J. et al; "Meal Timing and Composition Influence Ghrelin Levels, Appetite Scores and Weight Loss Maintenance in Overweight and Obese Adults," *Steroids,* 2011. doi: 10.1016/j.steroids.2011.12.006.

2. Schlundt, D.G. et al; "The Role of Breakfast in the Treatment of Obe-sity: A Randomized Clinical Trial," *Am J Clin Nutr,* 1992; 55:645–51.

3. O'Connor, A.; "Myths Surround Breakfast and Weight," *New York Times,* Sept. 10, 2013.

4. Ibid.

Chapter 23

1. "How Often Are Your Cells Replaced?" www.sciencemuseum.org.uk /whoami/findoutmore/yourbody/whatdoyourcellsdo/howoften areyourcellsreplaced.aspx.

2. Dossey, L.; "Shared, Rented, Occupied: Expanding Our Concept of Who We Are," *Explore,* Nov/Dec 2013; 9(6):339–343. http://download.journals.elsevierhealth.com/pdfs /journals/1550-8307/PIIS1550830713002462.pdf.

3. Feltman, R.; "The Gut's Microbiome Changes Rapidly with Diet: A New Study Finds That Populations of Bacteria in the Gut Are Highly Sensitive to the Food We Digest," *Scientific American,* Dec. 14, 2013.

4. Love, S.; "Risk Factors: Does Alcohol Increase Breast Cancer Risk?" www.dslrf.org/breastcancer/content.asp?CATID=60&L2=1&L3=6&L4 =0&PID=&sid=132&cid=596.

5. Ibid.

Chapter 25

1. Bishayee, A. et al; "Triterpenoids as potential agents for the chemopre vention and therapy of breast cancer," *Front Biosci,* Jan 1, 2011; 16: 980–996. Published online Jan 1, 2011.

2. Shanmugam, M. et al.; "Targeted inhibition of tumor proliferation, survival, and metastasis by pentacyclic triterpinoids: potential role in prevention and therapy of cancer," *Cancer Letters,* July 2012; 320(2):158–70. doi: 10.1016/j.canlet.2012.02.037.

3. Muraki, I. et al.; "Fruit consumption and risk of type 2 diabetes: results from three prospective longitudinal cohort studies," *BMJ,* published online August 29, 2013.

4. Franz, M.; "Your Brain on Blueberries: Enhance Memory with the Right Foods," *Scientific American,* Jan/Feb 2011. www.scientificamerican.com/article/your-brain-on-blueberries.

5. Katz, D.; "Unscrambling Egg Science," Huffington Post, 08/21/12. www.huffingtonpost.com/david-katz-md/eggs-health_b_1818209 .html.

6. Grzanna, R. et al; "Ginger: An Herbal Medicinal Product with Broad Anti-Inflammatory Actions," *J. Med Food,* 2005; 8(2):125–32.

7. Gruenwald, J. et al; "Cinnamon and Health," *Crit Rev Sci Nutri,* 2010; 50(9): 822–34. www.ncbi.nlm.nih.gov/pubmed/20924865.

8. "Hot Pepper Compound Could Help Hearts," *Science Daily,* March 27, 2012. www.sciencedaily.com/releases/2012/03/120327215605.htm.

9. Parker-Pope, T.; "The Science of Chicken Soup," http://well.blogs .nytimes.com/2007/10/12/the-science-of-chicken-soup/?_r=0.

Chapter 26

1. EWG's 2013 Shopper's Guide to Pesticides in Produce: www.ewg.org /foodnews/summary.php.

2. Ibid.

3. Dockterman, E.; "Food Waste Is Ripe for Profit," *Time,* Nov. 25, 2013.

Chapter 27

1. Rosenberg, D.; "Diet Advice from Israel: Eat Your Vegetables," 3/07/12. www.jpost.com/Health-and-Science/Diet-advice-from-Israel-Eat -your-vegetables.

2. Canfi, A. et al; "Effect of Changes in the Intake of Weight of Specific Food Groups on Successful Body Weight Loss During a Multi–Dietary Strategy Intervention Trial," *Journal of the American College of Nutrition,* 2011; 30(6):491–501.

3. Falalyeyeva, T.M. et al.; "Effect of Glyprolines on Homeostasis of Gastric Mucosa in Rats with Stress Ulcers," *Exp Biol Med,* 2010 Jul; 149(1) :26–8.

Acknowledgments

Think of the credits rolling by at the end of a motion picture, the audience so enthralled by the plot and the acting that they're still glued to their seats. The producers, writers and directors, stars and gaffers, cameramen and caterers . . . the list is so delightful because everyone gets their due. I've listed just a few of the cast who helped get this book out of my head (finally) and into your hands.

Whether they're doctors, nurses, nutritionists, editors, or psychologists, or poodles, spouse, or friend, every one has been integral—and indispensable—to the writing of this book.

This was a complex book to write, taking me into territory where I'd never been before. I've tried to synthesize an enormous amount of information for you—a daunting task, believe me—and I'm bound to have gone off track here and there. All the mistakes—and I'm sure there will be some—are mine alone. I absolve all the people whose work I've quoted and whose shoulders I stand upon.

I'm very grateful for the work of breakthrough thinkers whose work I admire, but many of whom I've never met. These include Gary Taubes; Michael Pollan; Dean Ornish, M.D.; Peter Attia, M.D.; Christopher Gardner, Ph.D.; Jeff Leach; Steven Gundry, M.D.; Robert Atkins, M.D.; David Katz, M.D.; William Davis, M.D.; and Chris Kresser.

Thanks to Michael Nova, M.D., and Sara Gottfried, M.D., for introducing me to the world of genetic testing.

And a very special thanks to David Perlmutter, M.D., who so graciously wrote the Foreword to this book when he was still on tour with his own book, *Grain Brain*. Special thanks as well to my friend Arielle Ford who connected us.

And now, let's roll the credits for the rest of *The PlantPlus Diet Solution* cast. I am so very grateful to:

Executive Producer: Louise Hay
Producer: Reid Tracy
Script: Joan Borysenko, Ph.D.
Director: Gordon Dveirin, Ed.D.
Canine Support: Milo and Mitzi
Editorial: Hay House Editorial
Cover: Steve Williams
Design: Riann Bender
Marketing: Richelle Zizian and Erin Dupree

Team Joanie: Thanks to all these good friends who shared information, inspiration, meals, recipes, laughter, and, in many cases, some very good red wine. You all know why I'm so very grateful to you:

- Christine Hibbard, Ph.D.
- David Hibbard, M.D.
- Sara Davidson
- Marilyn Tam
- Karen Drucker
- Lee McCormick
- Mee Tracy McCormick
- Angela Thomas, R.N.
- Keith Bell, L.Ac.
- Josh Sessions
- Ruth Buczynski, Ph.D.

- Pamela Peeke, M.D.

- Andrew Weil, M.D.

- James Gordon, M.D.

- Christiane Northrup, M.D.

- Martha Howard, M.D.

- Oriah Mountain Dreamer

- Larry Dossey, M.D.

- Loretta LaRoche

- Roger Jahnke, O.M.D.

- Nathaniel Kirkland, M.D.

. . . and the many research scientists whose work I've cited throughout the text. I'm fairly certain that I've left out some folks who deserve mention. If that's you, please forgive me. I'll cook a meal for you as penance.

About the Author

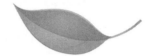

Joan Borysenko, Ph.D., and her husband, Gordon Dveirin, Ed.D., live high in the front range of the Rocky Mountains. Their mantra is *Outside!,* which suits their two standard poodles, Mitzi and Milo, just fine. Joan is a Harvard Medical School–trained cancer cell biologist, a licensed psychologist, and a *New York Times* best-selling author.

A pioneer in psychoneuroimmunology, mind-body medicine, and stress management, Joan is known for her tender exploration of the human spirit—what kindles it and what snuffs it out. President of Mind-Body Health Sciences, LLC, in Boulder, Colorado, she is a perennially popular national speaker and the author or co-author of 16 books. Joan's work has appeared in newspapers ranging from the *Washington Post* to the *Wall Street Journal,* as well as online in the Huffington Post, Oprah.com, and numerous other hubs.

Website: www.joanborysenko.com

Hay House Titles of Related Interest

YOU CAN HEAL YOUR LIFE, the movie, starring Louise Hay & Friends
(available as a 1-DVD program and an expanded 2-DVD set)
Watch the trailer at: www.LouiseHayMovie.com

THE SHIFT, the movie,
starring Dr. Wayne W. Dyer
(available as a 1-DVD program and an expanded 2-DVD set)
Watch the trailer at: www.DyerMovie.com

∅ ∅ ∅

ALL IS WELL: Heal Your Body with Medicine, Affirmations, and Intuition,
by Louise Hay and Mona Lisa Schulz, M.D., Ph.D.

CRAZY SEXY KITCHEN: 150 Plant-Empowered Recipes to Ignite a
Mouthwatering Revolution, by Kris Carr, with Chef Chad Sarno

MINDFUL LIVING, by Miraval

MIND OVER MEDICINE: Scientific Proof That You Can Heal Yourself,
by Lissa Rankin, M.D.

THE POWER OF SELF-HEALING: Unlock Your Natural Healing
Potential in 21 Days!, by Dr. Fabrizio Mancini

THE REAL FOOD REVOLUTION: Healthy Eating, Green Groceries, and the
Return of the American Family Farm, by Congressman Tim Ryan

All of the above are available at your local bookstore,
or may be ordered by contacting Hay House (see next page).

∅ ∅ ∅

We hope you enjoyed this Hay House book. If you'd like to receive our online catalog featuring additional information on Hay House books and products, or if you'd like to find out more about the Hay Foundation, please contact:

Hay House, Inc., P.O. Box 5100, Carlsbad, CA 92018-5100
(760) 431-7695 or (800) 654-5126
(760) 431-6948 (fax) or (800) 650-5115 (fax)
www.hayhouse.com® • www.hayfoundation.org

∅ ∅ ∅

Published and distributed in Australia by:
Hay House Australia Pty. Ltd., 18/36 Ralph St., Alexandria NSW 2015
Phone: 612-9669-4299 • *Fax:* 612-9669-4144 • www.hayhouse.com.au

Published and distributed in the United Kingdom by:
Hay House UK, Ltd., Astley House, 33 Notting Hill Gate, London W11 3JQ
Phone: 44-20-3675-2450 • *Fax:* 44-20-3675-2451 • www.hayhouse.co.uk

Published and distributed in the Republic of South Africa by:
Hay House SA (Pty), Ltd., P.O. Box 990, Witkoppen 2068
Phone/Fax: 27-11-467-8904 • www.hayhouse.co.za

Published in India by: Hay House Publishers India,
Muskaan Complex, Plot No. 3, B-2, Vasant Kunj, New Delhi 110 070
Phone: 91-11-4176-1620 • *Fax:* 91-11-4176-1630 • www.hayhouse.co.in

Distributed in Canada by:
Raincoast Books, 2440 Viking Way, Richmond, B.C. V6V 1N2
Phone: 1-800-663-5714 • *Fax:* 1-800-565-3770 • www.raincoast.com

∅ ∅ ∅

Take Your Soul on a Vacation

Visit www.HealYourLife.com® to regroup, recharge, and reconnect with your own magnificence. Featuring blogs, mind-body-spirit news, and life-changing wisdom from Louise Hay and friends.

Visit www.HealYourLife.com today!